PALEO
Easy As
1-2-3:

Lose Weight, Eat Great

Over 100 Dairy Free, Gluten Free, Grain Free Recipes | No Sugar or Salt Added

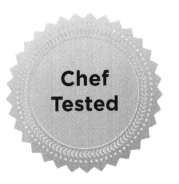

Chef Tested

By Donna Leahy

Paleo Easy as 1-2-3: Lose Weight, Eat Great

Food Arts Fusion LLC

© 2014, Donna Leahy

Disclaimer

The information contained in this book is based on research and personal experience unless otherwise stated. It should not be substituted for qualified medical advice. Health related information provided in this book is for educational and entertainment purposes only. Always seek the counsel of a qualified medical practitioner for an individual consultation before making any significant changes to your diet and lifestyle and to answer questions about specific medical conditions. The author and publisher disclaim responsibility for any adverse effects that may result from the use or application of the recipes and information within this book. The publisher and the author make no representations or warranties with respect to accuracy or completeness of the contents of this work and specifically disclaim all warranties including, without limitation, warranties of fitness, health or weight loss for a particular purpose. This is work is sold with the understanding that the publisher and author are not engaged in rendering medical or other professional advice and neither is liable for damages arising from it.

Table of Contents

Chapter 3

Chapter 4

Chapter 5

Chapter 6

Chapter 7

Chapter 8

Chapter 9

Chapter 1
Paleo Easy as 1-2-3

- Welcome to the Paleo Lifestyle!
- Why Easy as 1-2-3?
- Why Paleo?
- The Basics of Paleo
- Lists of Food Included and Not Included
- Fruits and Vegetables
- No Dairy Allowed
- Desserts, Sugar and Paleo Baking
- To Salt or not to Salt
- Alcohol and Its Effect on Metabolism
- Get Ready to Shop: Choosing Your Food
- Sample Week of Menus

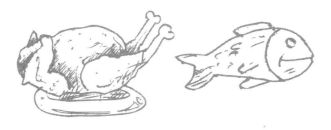

Welcome to the Paleo Lifestyle!

Paleo Easy As 1-2-3 is a simple plan to have you eat well and eat healthier foods at the same time. If you are new to Paleo, you will get started on the road to eating less processed food and enjoying delicious meals. If you're a seasoned Paleo follower, you will increase your eating pleasure with new creative recipes that make eating healthy easy and enjoyable.

Sometimes referred to as the Stone Age, Primal, Caveman or Hunter-Gatherer Diet, the basis of the Paleolithic way of eating is simple. Before processed food, people relied on whole foods – that is, foods as they appear in nature - for sustenance and energy. Once processed food became the mainstay of our eating, sugar and grains became central to what we eat. Advocates of the Paleo lifestyle argue that these carbohydrates are not what nature intended for us to eat. Farmed foods and food processing created an unhealthy lifestyle. So, to return to healthy eating, you need to follow a diet similar to what cavemen ate.

It's important for our health that we make our own choices about what's in the food we eat. But being selective about what we eat does not mean we can't have great tasting food. This is the first book in a series dedicated to creating wholesome meals that taste great.

I am an expert chef with a keen interest in encouraging people to prepare their own food. I know how to cook well, choose the best ingredients available, create tasty dishes and write recipes that work. I am also a published cookbook author. When my first cookbooks were published, I was the executive chef and owner of an award-winning country inn. Those cookbooks were, to a great extent, about me. They told my story through recipes and anecdotes. The photos featured my cuisine, presented the way I chose to plate it.

But this book is not about me. If you're interested in eating well and eating healthy, this book is written for you. You won't see before and after photos of people eating Paleo. You won't see photos of me cooking or even of the food I prepare. As a matter of fact, I've chosen not to include photos for a reason. I want this book to be about you participating in your path to better health – cooking wholesome dishes, enjoying what you eat and looking forward to preparing great meals. I want you to use these recipes to tell your story – a story about eating better and enjoying food more. I want you to personalize the recipes and present them in a way that pleases you. In short, I want you to enjoy cooking them. And of course, I want you to enjoy eating them too.

We've become a society of food voyeurs. We like to watch other people cook. There is evidence that we spend more time watching cooking shows than we do actually cooking. The cookbooks we spend top dollar on are "coffee table" books, featuring gorgeous photographs of the recipes and designed to stay out of the kitchen. Many of the most popular cooking blogs include beautifully styled photos of the food discussed. There is even a phrase to describe this – food porn. It's pervasive, especially on the Internet and in social media. How pervasive? Let's see. I just Googled the phrase and got about 143,000,000 results in 0.24 seconds. That pervasive.

Somehow cooking has become removed from our daily activity. We as a society no longer participate in preparing the food we eat, so it's no wonder we eat so much processed food. We eat out a lot too. Of course, I am not lobbying for you to never eat out again. (After all, I owned a restaurant!) And I also want you to enjoy all types of cookbooks (my previously published books featured beautiful photography). But my main goal here is to help you begin making better choices and participating in your food preparation. Like so many things in our passive lifestyle, we need to stop watching and start doing. We need to cultivate a culture of cooking. We need to place it at the top of our list, like many of us do with a daily workout at the gym, surfing the Internet or however we spend our extra time.

Why Easy as 1-2-3?

Through years of experience, I've come to believe that eating well and eating healthy go hand in hand. Both can be accomplished through three easy steps:

1) Limit consumption of processed food by cooking food ourselves.
2) Seek out high-quality, fresh ingredients from a trusted source.
3) Use recipes for creating delicious, healthy meals that are simple to execute.

As a professional chef, I have spent countless hours creating delicious dishes. The operative word her is "creating." Not cutting and pasting, not reordering ingredients – actually getting into the kitchen and coming up with fresh, interesting dishes. And then figuring out how those dishes can be turned out consistently. That's where expertise and a passion for good food come together. Creating food that tastes great and using quality ingredients is not just the domain of a professional chef. It's possible for everyone. It's the basis of good habits that can help you lead a healthier life.

Recently I was watching a television commercial for a well-known prepackaged diet plan. I suddenly realized what bothered me so much about it (other than the fact that the food looked terrible). Why would anyone give over the responsibility of preparing their food to a corporation? Why would they accept that it's better to eat a commercially prepared meal in a box than one created in their own kitchen? The answer is tragically simple: It seems easy – easy to let someone else make the decisions, easy to let someone else add they want to add, easy to let someone else package it to make it shelf stable and attractive.

You may be thinking, "Easy is good, right? I LIKE easy!" Maybe it's what attracted you to this book (which I am grateful for). So what's the trade-off? This answer is simple too: your health. By choosing processed foods in any form, you trade your health. Did you realize that's what you were doing when you wandered down the frozen food aisle looking for "easy?" I would guess you never really thought about it. Today I want to encourage you to start thinking about "easy" in a different light. It will change your life. What you're about to find out is that it can also be easy to eat well and eat healthy – it just takes a plan.

How did this happen to us? One could argue that the convenience foods of the '50s started a trend for prepackaged foods that led us to where we are today, and perhaps there is some truth to that. But I can tell you that, growing up in the '60s, I almost never ate prepackaged foods as a kid. My mom cooked. Sometimes we wished we could be the cool kids and have TV dinners! But we didn't prevail. I won't say we never had any food from a box or jar or can. But for the most part, we did not. Part of it was economics: Cooking from scratch was cheaper. And part of it was that my mom wanted to know what she was feeding us. Thank you, Mom.

I see moms (and dads) today wanting the same for their kids. I watch them check labels and study nutritional information – and all of that is a good start. But that's all it is. We need to move to a place where most of our food does not come with a label. Where it doesn't come in a box, bag or jar (even one made from recycled materials)! Check your grocery cart next time you're at the store. If the majority of the food in there doesn't have a label, you're on the right path. Otherwise, it's time to reconsider.

Cooking our meals is nothing new. In fact, it's as old as our species. It's been argued that the invention of cooking is what led to the rise of humanity. Fire freed us up to do other things. Our brains grew in size. We spent less time chewing and more time doing! We can get there again – we just have to make the effort and conscious choice. Like any other habit, it will become easier over time. And eventually it will simply become what we do!

Why Paleo?

The Paleo lifestyle is extremely popular and supports the culture of cooking. Paleo followers want to limit processed food in their diets and use wholesome sources for the meat and fish they consume. That's a big part of beginning down the path to a healthier life. So my plan is simple: Let's start with Paleo in its true form and create some recipes that will make us look forward to eating. Let's use the eating plan behind the Paleo movement to prove that no matter what restrictions we want to place on our eating – whether by choice (for reasons of fitness or healthy living) or by necessity (as in the case of those with allergies or digestive issues) – we can still eat well by preparing wholesome meals at home.

Of course, there are many people claiming to promote the Paleo lifestyle who include ingredients that really aren't part of the plan. There are also recipes that claim to promote "healthier" versions of ingredients that are not included in the Paleo plan. After seeing a host of different versions of what's allowed and what is not, I chose to use a strict interpretation of Paleo. By limiting ingredients, you will have the option to make additions as you see fit.

It's important to cut through the maze of misinformation regarding nutrition and find the facts. But doing so can be time consuming. When possible, I've tried to narrow it down to the facts so that you don't have to. In the end, everyone is responsible for their own health. You will need to make your own choices about how strict you will be in following the plan. In the recipes that follow, I've done some of that homework for you. So let's get started.

The Basics of Paleo

Millions of years ago we were hunter-gatherers. That bears some repeating – hunters AND gatherers. I wasn't there, but I would venture to say it was a lot easier to gather than to hunt. We ate lean meat, perhaps some fish, fresh fruits and vegetables. Recent scientific data indicates that as the Paleolithic diet was studied, it was originally overestimated just how much meat our ancestors consumed. Simply put, plant foods don't leave as clear of a record as meats do. (Common sense will tell you that as well.) Can you imagine how much meat you'd actually eat if you had to hunt it down, skin it and cook it over the campfire every time you got hungry? So just in case you're imagining that your new eating plan will have you mimicking the Hollywood caveman image of carrying around a giant brontosaurus leg to gnaw upon, put that image out of your mind. The majority of what our ancestors ate was more than likely NOT meat. While the Paleo plan does include lean meats and other lean proteins, at least half of what you consume should come from fruits and vegetables.

Let's take the thinking behind the Paleo lifestyle step by step. Our ancestors did not have access to the simple carbohydrates that are pervasive in the modern diet, like grains and sugar. Part of how we all survive is that our bodies metabolize the most accessible forms of energy first. In this manner, our bodies burn carbohydrates before fat because carbs burn more quickly. The human body relies heavily on stored carbohydrates as its main energy source. Fat must go through additional processes before being converted into energy. So in theory, eating excess carbs creates a readily available energy source. Instead of us eventually burning the fat we're storing in our bodies, we simply add to it.

The Paleo lifestyle changes this by doing one simple thing: removing many of the simple carbohydrates from your diet. This allows for something called lipolysis to occur. Lipolysis is the process of your body releasing fat stores to be burned as energy. So by reducing the available carbs, the Paleo plan allows your body to burn more fat. The simpler the carbohydrates, the quicker they turn into sugar and the more your body is prevented from burning fat. In fact, one of the main effects of overeating carbohydrates is that they simply replace fat as a source of energy.

But here's the thing – fat is a longer lasting and slower burning fuel than carbohydrates. Your body likes this! So when you stop eating simple carbohydrates and sugar, your body resorts to burning body fat for energy.

Due to some flawed research in the early 1960s, it became a common belief that saturated fat causes heart disease. In fact, we are now learning that sugar deserves more of the blame than fat. But there is definitely a point to be made about what kinds of fats we consume. Many nutrition experts believe that before we began to rely so heavily on processed foods, our Paleo ancestors consumed omega-3 and omega-6 fatty acids in roughly equal amounts. Anthropological research also suggests that our Paleo ancestors consumed omega-6 and omega-3 fats in a ratio of roughly 1:1. In our modern diet of processed foods, we now get far too much of the omega-6s and not enough of the omega-3s.

Without getting into the weeds here, omega-3 fats are anti-inflammatory while omega-6 fats are pro-inflammatory. We actually need both. Too much omega-3s and your blood will be too thin. Too much omega-6s may result in inflammation in your body. Elevated omega-6 intake is associated with an increase in all inflammatory diseases – including cardiovascular disease, type 2 diabetes, irritable bowel, rheumatoid arthritis, asthma, cancer and others.

One of the goals of the Paleo way of eating is to bring the omega-3s and 6s back into balance, especially by eliminating highly processed vegetable oils. So if we cut out some of those omega-6s by reducing consumption of processed and fast foods and polyunsaturated vegetable oils (corn, sunflower, safflower, soy and cottonseed, for example), and consume higher omega-3 foods like extra virgin olive oil, oily fish like salmon, walnuts and flax seeds, we limit inflammation and get our omega's back into balance. Seems simple, right?

So if it's so easy, why doesn't everyone follow it?

We all know the answer to this – taste! The biggest challenge to staying with any eating plan is enjoying the food we eat. That's where *Paleo Easy as 1-2-3* comes in. These are tested recipes that actually taste good. What, you say? What a concept! The whole concept of "diet" does not belong as part of a healthy eating plan. This is a permanent way to eat that is both healthy and enjoyable. Using the basis of the Paleo plan, these delicious meals will satisfy – and when you are satisfied, you don't seek out other options!

The first thing you will notice is that you will actually be required to prepare your own food. Don't let this scare you. These recipes have been developed for both ease of preparation and taste. If you need to lose weight, this plan will help you by reducing hunger and increasing satisfaction. You will be eating foods that are nutritiously whole. This may seem like a simple concept – and guess what? It is! We just need to get used to the idea that cooking is part of our path to improving our health. The good news is that, within the confines of the Paleo plan, you will be eating delicious, tasty foods – so much so that you won't have to think twice about heading into the kitchen to prepare your next meal. We'll also highlight recipes that can be made ahead of time so they can act as your new "convenience" food – no packaging required!

What makes this plan so easy is that it is simple – you won't have to count calories, measure foods or write down what you eat. Here's what you're going to be eating: lean meats, fish and poultry, fresh fruits and fresh non-starchy vegetables, eggs and nuts. Does this mean you will never eat any other ever again? Of course not. But the goal is for you to be happy eating these foods the majority of the time. We think that you will find that once you eliminate the sugar and starches of processed foods, you will not miss them as much as you think. And the longer you can do without them, the more likely you will be to never want to eat them again.

We're also going to concentrate on the quality of the foods you chose. This is where you are going to acquire the knowledge needed to make good choices about what you eat.

List of Food Included and Not Included

LIST OF WHAT IS INCLUDED

Here is a list of the ingredients you WILL find in these recipes:

- Meat (poultry and organ meat, including liver)
- Fish
- Healthy oils (olive, walnut, avocado, coconut, macadamia)
- All vegetables, except white potatoes
- All fruits
- Unsweetened coconut, full fat coconut milk and coconut cream
- Nuts and seeds (preferably raw and unsalted)
- Fresh herbs
- Spices without salt added
- Wine for cooking – optional

LIST OF WHAT'S NOT INCLUDED

Here is a basic list of ingredients that you will NOT find in these Paleo plan recipes:

- Any processed foods, included salt cured and pickled ones
- Grains, including cereal grains

- Legumes (i.e. beans and peanuts)
- Added salt in all forms, including cured meats like bacon
- Fruit juices, fresh or otherwise
- Refined vegetable oils
- Vinegar and other fermented foods, like fish sauce
- Soy
- Added sugar in all forms, including honey
- Dairy
- White potatoes

Fruits and Vegetables

In recent years, many of the high protein, high fat diets have encouraged people to lose weight by drastically limiting the amount of carbohydrates they consume. This has resulted in limiting fruits and vegetables, which are some of our most nutrient-dense foods. In the Paleo plan, you will be consuming carbohydrates in the form of fruits and vegetables. These mostly non-starchy carbs will help you feel satisfied and provide much-needed nutrients.

The idea that fruit is full of sugar needs to be put into perspective. Yes, when you eat fruit, the overwhelming majority of the calories you consume are supplied by carbohydrate – mostly in the form of fructose, which is the natural sugar in fruit. However, all plant foods are predominantly carbohydrate (in addition to structural elements, like cellulose, that provide fiber). When you eat vegetables, the majority of the calories you're eating come from carbohydrate, too. In the absence of added sugars (think brownies, pancakes with maple syrup, peanut butter and jelly) the natural sugar of fruits will provide the closest thing to "dessert" that you will find in a Paleo plan. The dessert recipes in this book are mostly fruit based and are not sweet in the sense that many of our palates have come to expect.

Some people argue that all fruits are not created equally. Some are actually quite a bit higher in natural sugars and may not be in line with the eating patterns of our Paleo ancestors. Part of this might be that modern agriculture has skewed the fruits grown towards the sugar-loving palate of our modern diet. Another part is perhaps that some fruits are just sweeter. Often the concept of how much a food increases blood glucose levels after eating (called the glycemic index) is used to encourage people to eat lower sugar fruit.

A newer concept, called glycemic load, also considers the portion size and the net carbohydrates in the fruit. When you take glycemic load into account, nearly all fruits (including pineapple and watermelon) and vegetables (including pumpkin) are acceptable. Fruits and veggies also provide the majority of the nutrients and fiber in your diet. Many Paleo experts recommend fruit with every meal. So again, use discretion but don't shy away from eating this healthy alternative to processed sweets.

Legumes and white potatoes are not included on the Paleo vegetable list. Legumes include beans (dried and fresh) and peanuts. Part of the basis for not allowing them is that legumes and potatoes contain antinutrients, compounds that reduce the body's ability to absorb and use essential nutrients. Potatoes are thought to cause intestinal permeability, commonly referred to as "leaky gut." However, there is some evidence to suggest that cooked legumes and potatoes are part of a healthy diet and were consumed by our ancestors. Again, this is an individual choice that everyone needs to make. However, in keeping true to the tenets of the Paleo lifestyle, none of the recipes will include legumes or white potatoes.

No Dairy Allowed

The Paleo lifestyle argues that our ancestors did not have domesticated cows to milk. In addition, consumption of dairy has been linked in some studies to diabetes. However, there are many Paleo followers who include some dairy, specifically pasture-raised, grass-fed, full fat and fermented dairy like yogurt and cheese. A specialized clarified butter called ghee (in which the milk solids are caramelized) is often included because it has a similar composition to other healthy saturated fats. Even butter made with milk from grass-fed cows is sometimes featured in recipes. But again, the Paleo way of eating does not include dairy, so you won't find it in these recipes.

Coconut milk is made by soaking grated white coconut and straining the resulting liquid. It does not contain dairy. Look for brands that are free of BPA (a chemical added to can linings) and guar gum (a natural gum that can cause intestinal upset) when possible. Guar gum also has a negative effect on the flavor of the coconut milk.

Desserts, Sugar and Paleo Baking

Paleo baking may seem like a misnomer. Did the cave people gather by the fire for waffles or cake? Probably not. However, a few recipes are included here to allow for an occasional baked dessert or breakfast treat. Paleo recipes typically include coconut flour and/or almond flour. Several recipes in this book utilize either of these two flours in lieu of wheat or other grain-based flours. However, there are some reasons to limit the consumption of baked goods and almond flour in particular.

Almond flour is nothing more than finely ground almonds. One ounce of almonds has approximately 23 nuts. So, doing the math, a cup of almond flour has the equivalent of over 90 nuts. That's a lot of nuts! The other concern with almond flour is that it contains high amounts of omega-6 fatty acids. As previously noted, omega-6 fatty acids are thought to cause increased inflammation. However, strictly speaking, almond flour and coconut flour conform to the list of ingredients widely accepted on Paleo. The real concern is over-consuming these recipes.

In keeping with the Paleo way of eating, there is no added sugar in any of these recipes (fruit is often used instead, but still without adding sugar). You may find that these recipes (mainly baked desserts and a few breakfast items like pancakes) are not sweet. Experts argue that our palate is used to consuming an average of 18–25 teaspoons of added sugar per day, so cutting back to zero added sugar may be quite a shock. Some Paleo recipes included maple syrup or honey as sweeteners. But, strictly speaking, added sugar in any form is not allowed on Paleo so these recipes do not include it. Here is another instance when it's up to you to make a choice. If you decide to add maple syrup or honey to any of the recipes, just do it with the knowledge that these so-called "healthy" sweeteners are still added sugar.

So why include these recipes? Even without the added sugar, the recipes for pancakes and desserts are tasty and satisfying. Consumed in moderation, these recipes may make it easier for you to stick with the overall Paleo plan.

To Salt or Not to Salt

Salt in the form of sodium chloride is essential to maintain fluid balance, transmit signals in our nervous systems and help regulate blood pressure. Our bodies need it. Salt does occur naturally at low levels in all foods. However, processed foods typically include excessive amounts of added salt. By eliminating processed foods, Paleo also eliminates a hidden source of salt. Studies show that salt is an acquired taste. So why is a sprinkle of table salt not allowed on Paleo?

The theory is that Paleolithic diets were very low in sodium. There is evidence that our Paleo ancestors did not add salt to their food. Some in the Paleo community believe that the chloride in table salt can create an acidic load on your kidneys. Your body needs to be in a slightly alkaline environment to be at its healthiest, so the theory is that by eliminating added salt (along with consuming more alkaline foods like fruits and vegetables) your body will become more alkaline. However, there is opposing evidence arguing that reducing salt too much can actually harm our health. Again, here is another area where you will need to make a choice of when and if to add salt. But in keeping with the Paleo plan, the recipes here do not have table salt as an ingredient.

Baking soda (sodium bicarbonate) is chemically different from table salt. Baking soda is used in some of the recipes, including desserts and breakfast goods like pancakes. The bicarbonate part of baking soda neutralizes acids. It is used here as a leavening agent.

Alcohol and Its Effect on Metabolism

The Paleo lifestyle includes the option for moderate alcohol consumption (primarily red wine and some distilled spirits). In the recipes that follow, alcohol (mainly in the form of wine) is used to enhance cooking flavor (where, in fact, the alcohol is actually burned off). This addition will always be optional and can be replaced by chicken or beef stock in most cases. Whether or not to consume alcohol in any form as part of this plan is a personal choice that you will need to make. However, if part of your goal with Paleo is to lose weight, it is important to remember that drinking alcohol is sometimes counterproductive to weight loss. Here's why.

As already mentioned, the type of fuel your body uses is dictated to some extent by availability. That is, your body will burn the most readily available fuel. When alcohol is introduced into your system, it bumps up to the front of the metabolic line. When we go out for a night of drinking, our bodies will burn up the alcohol first. At the risk of oversimplifying the process, a small portion of alcohol is converted into fat and the rest is converted by your liver into acetate. Your body will metabolize the acetate first. The way your body responds to alcohol is very similar to the way it deals with excess carbohydrate.

Many carbohydrates are stored as a backup source of energy in the liver and muscles called glycogen. Thankfully, alcohol is not. Therefore, your body will return immediately to a fat burning state once the alcohol is used up. But how long that takes is directly related to how much is consumed. In this way, weight loss may still be achieved (or weight gain avoided) if alcohol consumption is done in moderation (and as long as you are burning more fat than you are putting on).

Get Ready to Shop: Choosing Your Food

Let's talk a little bit about food quality. Again, it's quite simple. Here are a few worthy goals to strive for whenever possible.

- Buy local.
- Buy fresh.
- Grow your own.
- Choose free range, grass fed and wild caught.
- Prepare everything yourself.

Why local? In short, because you can personally see how the products are being grown. Yes, it's harder to do this when you live in a major metropolitan area. But the real point is accountability. Now that you are taking responsibility for what's in the food you eat, buying some or any of those ingredients locally adds another layer of personal control over what you put into your body. Are there other farmers out there with integrity who are not local? Of course. And let's face it – we may not be able to get everything we eat locally. We may need to rely on the integrity of those farmers. But whenever there is an option to not rely on someone else when it comes to our food choices, let's make that our first priority.

Now you're thinking, "I have to spend time cooking, and now going from farm to farm for my ingredients? How am I going to work this into my already crammed schedule?" One option is to participate in Community Supported Agriculture (CSA). Basically you make an agreement with local farmers to support their production in exchange for a share of it. Typically there are drop-off points set up. (In the company's efforts to support local farmers, Whole Foods locations will act as a drop-off point for a CSA if there is a demand.) But some CSA's also offer delivery. If you decide to go this route, take some time to explore what options are available and if they suit your needs. It's always worthwhile to visit the farm locations personally and get feedback from other members to see if they are satisfied with the service.

The same idea applies when it comes to buying fresh. There is much less opportunity for someone to get between our food and us when it's fresh. Frozen produce from a local source may also be a good second option – just keep it as close to fresh and local as possible.

If you have the opportunity to grow some of your own produce, the experience will alter your life. I'm serious! There is something amazing about walking out to your garden and plucking a fresh vegetable right from the vine. Even in more urban areas, there are community gardens springing up that allow you the opportunity to experience this. And no matter where you live, you can always grow your own herbs. Choose a planter or a group of smaller pots that will fit into the area you have available. Add some potting mix and plants, and place them on your windowsill or under a grow light. Then start snipping! It's that easy.

Now for the somewhat daunting topic of choosing free range, grass fed and wild caught. There is not a lot to say here that won't be contested by one camp or another, so let's keeps this simple. If you can afford making these choices (and yes, these can be expensive food choices), you may be happier with the quality of the food and the added nutritional content. It may make you feel happier to know that the animals you are consuming as food were well treated and allowed to eat a natural diet. You may enjoy eating a wild caught fish instead of one that has been farm raised. All of these subjects are open to debate.

One fact that cannot be argued is that cattle, cows and chickens do not eat soy and corn naturally. Another fact is that many organic meats are fed soy and corn. And yet another fact is that wild game (think venison, bison, rabbit, etc.) has leaner meat, a lower content of omega-6 fatty acids and a higher content of omega-3 fatty acids. This is also true of grass fed animals in general. (Remember that too much omega-6 may result in inflammation in your body and is associated with an increase in all inflammatory diseases.)

So where does that leave us? With more choices to make. The fact that we are thinking about where our food comes from and making informed choices is really what matters most. The good thing is that making many of these choices will add to your eating satisfaction. Personally I find the eggs from free range chickens are awesomely delicious. Adding wild game to your diet adds variety and some really tasty eating options. I prefer wild caught fish mostly because I think they taste better. I would prefer the animals I consume to be treated well. But that's just me. That being said, part of the Paleo lifestyle is to make these choices your own.

Is it easier to gradually eliminate processed foods and simple carbohydrates, or to go cold turkey? It's different for everyone, so you might choose to do this plan 100% or incrementally. You might also go along with a partial plan, where you eat Paleo most of the time but allow yourself some days where you are not as strict. Whatever you decide, try to keep in mind the why behind the what. Remember that the most basic tenet is to stop eating processed foods.

Sample Week of Menus

The purpose of these recipes is to offer ideas and strategies for making delicious meals. They are scaled to serve four, so you can easily double the number of servings for more portions. In some cases, you can also divide the recipes for fewer portions. If you are eating on your own, it might be a good idea to befriend a fellow Paleo eater and share meals when you make extra. You may add as many recipes to your daily routine as you see fit. The sample weekly menu below includes 1–2 dishes per day from the recipes for weekdays (days 1–5) and several on weekends (Days 6–7). Day 7 is an example of what you might prepare if you were having guests for dinner. You will need to customize this so that it works with your schedule and demands. Feel free to add recipes on days when you have the time and interest in making them, or remove them from days when you don't.

Day 1

Breakfast: Omelet with scallions and mushrooms. Fresh fruit.

Lunch: Crab and Avocado Salad (see p. 103).

Snack: Mixed nuts.

Dinner: Roasted chicken with vegetables. Fresh fruit.

Day 2

Breakfast: Salmon Frittata (see p. 61).

Lunch: Leftover chicken with salad and walnuts.

Snack: Fresh fruit

Dinner: Broiled fish with vegetables. Fresh fruit

Day 3

Breakfast: Scrambled eggs with herbs. Fresh fruit.

Lunch: Grilled tuna with salad.

Snack: Roasted Eggplant Dip (see p. 80) with carrot sticks.

Dinner: Seared hamburger with vegetables. Fresh fruit.

Day 4

Breakfast: Mix of fresh fruit with toasted coconut flakes and nuts.

Lunch: Chicken breast with salad.

Snack: Spiced Nuts (see p. 87).

Dinner: Shrimp with Almonds and Mango Salsa (see p. 118).

Day 5

Breakfast: Poached eggs with salsa. Fresh fruit.

Lunch: Asparagus Soup (see p. 111).

Snack: Smoked fish.

Dinner: Grilled steak with salad and sweet potato.

Day 6

Breakfast: Cinnamon Crepes with Berries (see p. 74).

Lunch: Egg salad in lettuce leaves.

Snack: Lemon Pepper Crackers (see p. 84) and Green Vegetable Dip (see p. 95).

Dinner: Roasted pork loin with baked apples. Roasted Brussels Sprouts (see p. 153).

Day 7

Breakfast: Avocado Eggs Benedict (see p. 76).

Lunch: Salad with tomatoes, carrots and mushrooms. Fresh fruit.

Starter/Snack: Chicken Liver Pate (see p. 88).

Dinner: Buffalo Chili with Butternut Squash (see p. 132).

Dessert: Roasted Pears with Almond Crumble (see p. 174).

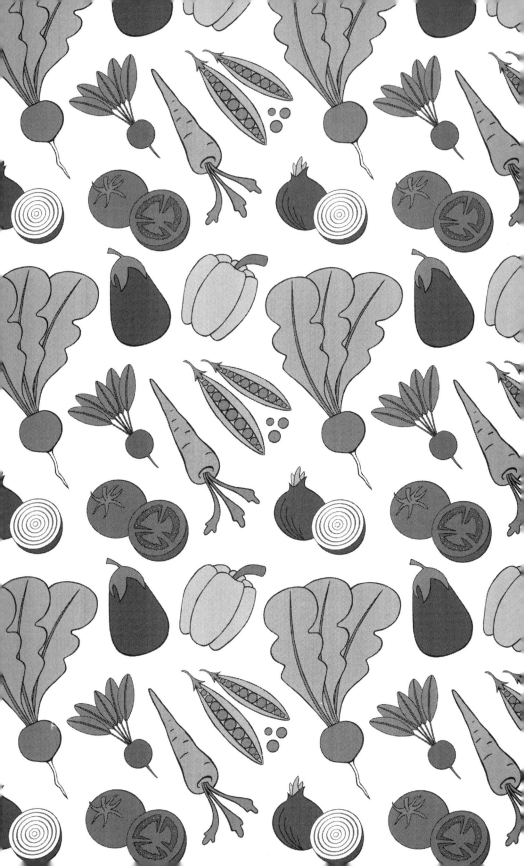

Chapter 2

Techniques and Tools

Techniques

Blanching

Roasting

Toasting Nuts

Making Ice Cream and Sorbet

How to Poach an Egg

Tools

Knives

Garlic Press

Citrus Press

Microplane Grater

Vegetable Peeler

Instant-read and Meat Thermometer

Food Processor

Blender

Cast Iron Dutch Oven

Ice Cream Maker

Ramekins

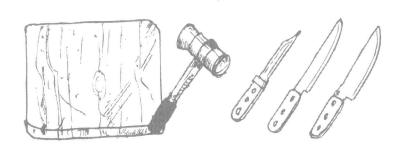

Techniques

Blanching

Blanching brightens the color of green vegetables and allows them to retain their color without turning brown as they cook (this is often referred to as "fixing" the color). It also allows them to retain a crisp texture when cooked. It can also be used to prepare fresh fruits and vegetables for storage in the freezer. Blanching food before freezing helps to preserve it by destroying bacteria that causes food to spoil, and also prevents discoloration. This is especially important if you purchase fresh fruits and vegetables in bulk and want to avoid waste. Blanching can also be used to remove thin skins from tomatoes, peaches and other fruits. But generally blanching is used to prevent overcooking vegetables and to help retain their nutritional value.

Basically the vegetables or fruit are dropped into boiling water for a brief time, drained and then plunged into ice water to rapidly stop the cooking process. All blanching requires boiling water and an ice bath. Prepare the ice bath first so the water gets very cold. Fill a large bowl about halfway with ice and then fill with water. Also fill a pot or skillet with water and bring to a boil over high heat. (Typically water is heavily salted for blanching green vegetables, but since the Paleo plan does not allow salt, it's not used here.)

To fix the colors of green vegetables, place your vegetables into the boiling water. The water temperature will drop and then return to a boil. Once it returns to a boil, the vegetables will typically take less than three minutes. They should be crisp, yet slightly undercooked. Quickly remove them from the boiling water (either pour into a strainer or remove them with tongs into a strainer). Immediately plunge them into the ice bath.

If you'd like to serve fully cooked vegetables cold (for example, asparagus in a salad), simply extend the cooking time until the vegetable is cooked through. Then proceed to remove them from the boiling water and plunge them into the ice bath.

To remove the skin of tomatoes (or thin skinned fruits like peaches or plums), use a paring knife to cut a very shallow X on the bottom of the tomato. Drop the tomato into the boiling water. Remove it when the skin begins to peel, about 30–60 seconds. Immediately remove the tomato and submerge it into the prepared bowl of ice water. Allow it to cool in the ice water completely, about 5 minutes. This will ensure that the tomato (or fruit) does not continue cooking. Then remove the tomato and peel the skin off. (To remove the seeds, simply quarter the peeled tomato and use a spoon to remove them. If you are going to use the tomatoes in sauce and the shape does not matter, squeezing the seeds out is even simpler.)

Roasting

Roasting is a simple technique for bringing out the best in high quality poultry, meat and even vegetables. It requires little preparation and can yield a bounty of leftovers, perfect for meals on the go. Roasting is cooking with dry heat, so no moisture is added to the pan. Place the roasting pan in the center of the oven so the heat circulates evenly around it. Prepare the items for roasting by lightly coating them with oil and seasoning with freshly ground pepper. Add spices and herbs to taste.

Vegetables for roasting should be cut into approximately two-inch pieces. Roast them in a preheated 400 degree F. oven for 40–50 minutes until tender and lightly caramelized. Stir the vegetables to turn them every 15–20 minutes. Firm vegetables like carrots, sweet potatoes and onions can be added directly to the roasting pan with meat or poultry, approximately 45 minutes before the meat or poultry is done.

When roasting poultry or meat, use a meat thermometer. Insert the thermometer into the thickest part of the meat. A list of the USDA recommended temperatures can be found here: http://www.foodsafety.gov/keep/charts/meatchart.html

Toasting Nuts

Toasting nuts intensifies their flavor and makes them crisp.

Oven method: Preheat the oven to 325 degrees F. Spread the nuts in a single layer on a baking sheet with a rim. The nuts can go from toasted to burnt very quickly, so keep your attention on them for the next 5–10 minutes. Small nuts like pistachios will toast much faster than larger ones like walnuts.

Stove top method: Heat a medium skillet over medium heat. Add the nuts and stir constantly to avoid dark spots. Nuts will be lightly browned and smell fragrant when ready.

Making Ice Cream and Sorbet

Although an ice cream machine is on the list of tools, it is possible to make ice cream and other frozen treats without one. However, it will take longer and the texture may not be as smooth.

Begin by freezing the mixture for about 45–55 minutes, depending on your freezer and the temperature of the mixture (do not let it freeze solid). Stir it vigorously with a whisk (or beat with a hand mixer or immersion blender) then return it to the freezer. Repeat every 30 minutes for about 2–3 hours or until the mixture is frozen but able to be scooped.

How to Poach an Egg

The biggest tip I can give you about poaching eggs is to be bold. Don't be afraid of the process, as it's quite simple.

Use a medium skillet for four eggs or less. For more, use a large skillet, as it's important to not crowd the eggs. Fill the skillet with about 2 1/2 inches of water and bring the water to a boil. Then lower the heat until the water is at a simmer. Take a spoon and swirl it around the inner edge of the pan a few times to create a whirlpool effect. Work quickly to get the eggs into the water while the water is still swirling. Crack the first egg and then hold it very close to the water to allow it to slip in gently. Continue adding eggs as desired. Slide a slotted spoon under the egg to keep it from sticking to the bottom and to collect the egg white into a ball around the yolk. Cover the pan.

Three minutes after adding the first egg, slip a slotted spoon under it and remove it from the water. Roll it from side to side to allow water to drain off. Then gently roll the egg onto a paper towel to absorb any excess water, and slide the egg onto a plate. Repeat in the order that the eggs were added. (Note: A runny yolk will take three minutes. For well done, allow for four minutes.)

Lemons, Limes and Zesting

Since Paleo does not allow vinegar, lemon and lime juice will be one of the primary ways to add acid to various dishes. Acid creates balance in food, brightens the flavors and actually stimulates the palate.

The recipes assume you will always use freshly squeezed lemon or lime juice. A citrus juicer (see note under Tools) is a handy tool that will allow the juice to pass through without the seeds or pulp for most uses. If a larger quantity of lemon or lime juice is required, pour the juice through a mesh strainer before using to ensure it is completely free of pulp and seeds.

When a recipe calls for lemon or lime zest, use only the zest from fresh lemons or limes. Zest is the outermost rind of the citrus fruit. The aromatic oils in the rind add flavor without the bitterness of the inner part of the peel (called the pith). Using a Microplane grater (see Tools) is the simplest way to get freshly grated zest. To remove the coating of food grade wax used on many citrus fruits, pour on boiling hot water and scrub the exterior vigorously before zesting. Many organically grown lemons and limes are not wax coated.

Tools

Most of these recipes assume that you will have use of basic utensils such as wooden spoons, ladles, whisks, tongs and spatulas; cutting boards; strainers and bowls; a timer; saucepans; and skillets (including at least one PFOA free non-stick skillet).

Here is a list of additional equipment that will make cooking these recipes at home easier:

Knives

Knives are a worthwhile investment. Most quality brands offer a lifetime guarantee. They will honor it unless you've done something nasty to your knife (like try to pry something open and break off the tip – you know who you are!). So purchase a brand that carries a warranty. Do your research online before shopping but definitely go to a store that allows you to actually cut with the knife. It needs to be comfortable in your hand (everyone is different) and have balance. There are three knives that everyone needs: an eight- to nine-inch chef's knife (size depends on how comfortable the knife feels in your hand); a three- to four-inch paring knife (size also a comfort issue); and a serrated knife, typically called a bread knife. Use the serrated knife only when you need to cut across an item. Purchase a honing steel and ask for a demonstration of how to use it to keep your new knives in good condition.

Garlic Press

Seasoning is very important in Paleo so you will likely use a lot of fresh garlic. A good garlic press will mince unpeeled cloves and is easy to clean.

Citrus Press

Choose one that is big enough to juice both a lime and lemon. A ratchet design makes pressing require less effort.

Microplane Grater

This is one instance where a name brand really equals quality, so it's included here. Microplane (also known generically as a rasp grater) is invaluable for easily zesting lemons and limes and grating ginger and nutmeg.

Vegetable Peeler

Traditional peelers have a swivel design, which is perfect for peeling most vegetables. A Y-shaped peeler makes it easier to peel some larger veggies like winter squash. A julienne peeler is very handy if you plan to shred zucchini and other vegetables into spaghetti-like pieces.

Instant-read and Meat Thermometer

An instant-read thermometer is for all-purpose use when measuring temperatures. But a leave-in thermometer for larger cuts of meat is essential to not allowing them to lose their moisture by "poking" the meat, as you would with the instant-read.

Food Processor

Yes, it's possible to prepare food without one – but a food processor makes some jobs so much easier. If you need to chop a bunch of vegetables and they don't have to be uniformly cut, a food processor makes the job a breeze. It's also great for making salad dressings, mayonnaise and pesto, because the motor can be left on while the oil is drizzled in to form an emulsion.

Blender

"But I have a food processor," you say! Not so fast. A blender is a better choice for liquids, as the lid seals tight. Use caution if using a regular blender for hot liquids. Leave the lid cap off for steam to escape and hold a thick folded towel or hot pad over it. Only fill it half full, allowing more room for expansion. An immersion blender is also a good blending option, especially for hot liquids like soups.

Cast Iron Dutch Oven

If you haven't cooked with cast iron, you're missing out. Cast iron conducts heat evenly, goes from stovetop to oven and will help you roast the tastiest and moistest poultry and meat with ease. Le Creuset brand from France is a substantial investment but the enamel interior makes it easy to see what's cooking, even in a darker oven. It also carries a lifetime warranty. (Le Creuset refers to their cast iron as "French ovens.") However, Lodge and Staub also make high performing cast iron. If the price is a big deterrent, cast iron is often given up for next to nothing at tag sales and second-hand stores. A five- to six-qt. size is the most versatile.

Ice Cream Maker

The action of an ice cream maker creates a smaller crystal and thus a creamier texture. Since fresh fruit is the basis of many Paleo desserts, purchasing an ice cream maker to make frozen treats is a worthwhile investment. There is a wide range of machines priced to match any budget. The lower priced machines usually require freezing the bowl for 24 hours in advance, so they do require some preplanning.

However, it is possible to make ice cream or sorbet without a machine (although the texture might not be as smooth). (see Technique p. 34).

Ramekins

A ramekin is an individual baking dish, typically five to six oz. per serving. Custard cups of a similar size could be substituted. If you decide to use a larger baking dish instead, you will need to add baking time to make sure the dish is cooked through.

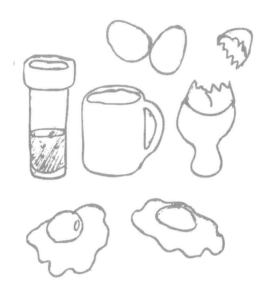

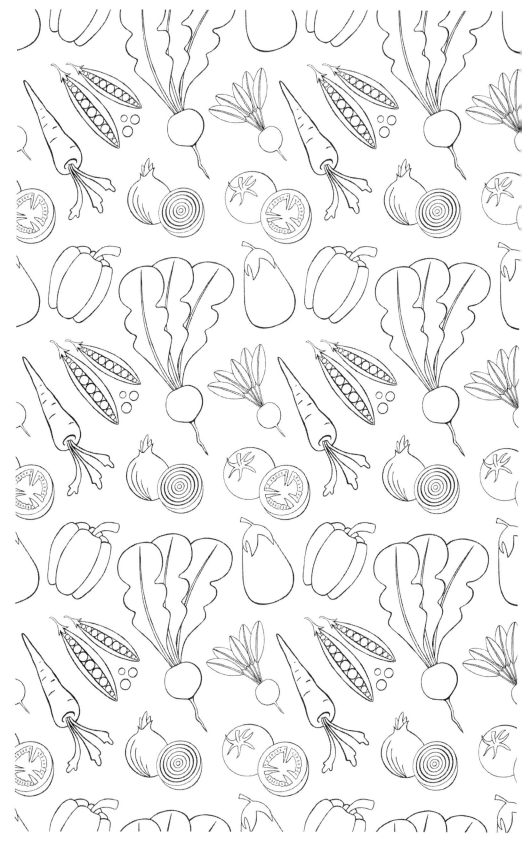

Chapter 3

Stocks and Pantry Basics

- Chicken Stock
- Beef Stock
- Fish Stock
- Pesto
- Tapenade
- Homemade Sausage

- Hollandaise
- Tomato Salsa
- Mayonnaise
- Salad Dressing
- Chili Powder

Chicken Stock
(aka Chicken Bone Broth)

The key to making stock or bone broth is to roast the bones before simmering and then simmer for an extended time (anywhere from 8 to 18 hours). Roasting will remove the fat (which can leave a greasy film) and develop a more complex flavor profile. The long simmering will render the gelatin from the bones, releasing nutrients like calcium and glucosamine chondroitin. The really important part is that it tastes complex and delicious. It also serves for the base of many dishes, adding levels of flavor not found in simple broths.

 Makes about 4 quarts

- 4 lbs. chicken bones, chopped into 3- to 4-inch pieces (or use 2 chicken carcasses from roasting)
- 2 cups onions, chopped into 2-inch pieces
- 1 cup celery, chopped into 2-inch pieces
- 1 cup carrots, chopped into 2-inch pieces
- ½ cup white wine (optional)
- 10 black peppercorns
- 2 bay leaves
- 3 sprigs fresh thyme

1. Preheat oven to 400 degrees F.

2. Combine chicken bones (or chopped carcasses), onions, celery, and carrots in a large roasting pan. Roast until the bones and vegetables are golden brown, about 30–40 minutes.

3. Pour off any grease and place the pan onto the stove top over medium high heat for 1–2 minutes until steaming. Remove the pan from the heat and quickly pour in the white wine (or use water). Return pan to heat. Bring liquid just to a boil and scrape off any brown bits into the liquid. Remove from heat and pour this mixture into a large stock pot. Add the peppercorns and herbs. Add 16 cups

of cold water. Bring the liquid up to a boil and reduce to a simmer. Cook for at least 8 hours. Skim off any foam and add water as necessary to keep bones submerged.

4. Remove from the heat and cool slightly. Strain the liquid through a sieve and discard the bones. Refrigerate until completely chilled through and gel-like in consistency. Skim off any fat that has risen to the surface and reserve for cooking if desired. Refrigerate for up to 1 week or freeze for up to 5 months.

Chef's Tip: Never throw out your roasted chicken carcass. If you don't have time to make stock that day, place it into a Ziploc bag and freeze it until ready to make stock. Allow the carcass to defrost in the refrigerator before using.

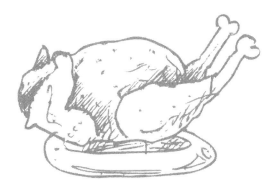

Beef Stock (aka Beef Bone Broth)

Freezing some stock in ice cube trays (and then storing the cubes in freezer bags) allows for easy portioning.

 Makes about 4 quarts

- 7 lbs. beef bones, sawed into 3-inch pieces if possible (ask your butcher to do this)
- 2 cups onions, chopped into 2-inch pieces
- 1 cup celery, chopped into 2-inch pieces

- 1 cup carrots, chopped into 2-inch pieces
- ¾ cup red wine (optional)
- 10 peppercorns
- 3 cloves garlic, peeled
- 3 bay leaves
- 2 sprigs fresh thyme

1. Preheat the oven to 400 degrees F.

2. Place the bones onto a roasting pan and roast for 1 hour. Remove from the oven. Lay the vegetables over the bones. Return to the oven and roast for 30 more minutes. Pour off any grease and place the pan onto the stove top over medium high heat for 1–2 minutes, until steaming. Remove the pan from the heat and quickly pour in the red wine (or use water). Return pan to heat. Bring liquid just to a boil and scrape off any brown bits into the liquid. Remove from heat and pour this mixture into a large stock pot. Add the peppercorns, garlic and herbs. Add 16 cups of water. Bring the liquid up to a boil and then reduce to a simmer. Cook for at least 8 and up to 18 hours. Skim off any foam and add water as necessary to keep bones submerged. Remove from the heat and cool slightly. Strain the liquid through a sieve and discard the bones. Refrigerate until completely chilled through and gel-like in consistency. Skim off any fat that has risen to the surface. Refrigerate for up to 1 week or freeze for up to 5 months.

Chef's Tip: Having the beef bones sawed into smaller pieces by your butcher will cut down on the cooking time.

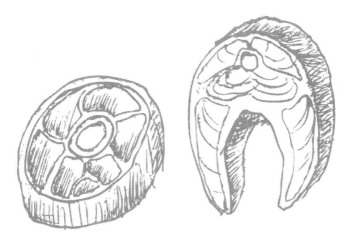

Fish Stock

Fish stocks add flavor to fish soups and other dishes and are a good use for leftover bones. This is not a bone broth in the sense that you don't roast the bones or cook them down (there's no marrow). Unlike chicken or beef, fish stocks are not cooked for more than 25 minutes or they can become bitter tasting. The vegetables are cut into smaller pieces to accommodate the shorter cooking time.

 Makes 2 quarts

- 2 tbsps. extra virgin olive oil
- 1 cup coarsely chopped leeks, white part only
- 1 cup onion, chopped into ¼-inch pieces
- 1 cup carrots, chopped into ¼-inch pieces
- 1 cup celery, chopped into ¼-inch pieces
- ½ bulb fennel, trimmed and chopped into ¼-inch pieces
- 4 lbs. heads and bones of non-oily white fish, such as sole, flounder, snapper or sea bass
- 1 cup dry white wine (optional)
- 8 whole black peppercorns
- 2 bay leaves
- 6 sprigs fresh thyme

1. Heat olive oil in a large stockpot over medium heat. Add the leek, onion, carrots, celery, and fennel bulb; cook until vegetables are tender, 8–10 minutes. Increase heat to medium high, then add fish heads and bones. Cook stirring constantly for 5 minutes. Add wine if using. Stir in the peppercorns and herbs. Add 12 cups of cold water. Bring liquid to a boil. Reduce heat to low and simmer 25 minutes, skimming any scum that rises to the surface. Turn off the heat and let cool slightly.

2. Strain the stock through a fine sieve set over a medium bowl. If you are not going to be using the stock within the hour, chill it as quickly as possible. Prepare an ice bath by filling a large bowl with ice and water.

Set the bowl of stock in the ice bath and allow the stock to cool. Cover the stock after it has completely cooled and keep refrigerated for up to 3 days, or freeze for up to 2 months.

Chef's Tip: Ask your fishmonger to save the heads and bones from filets for use in stock.

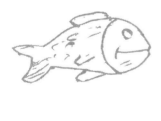
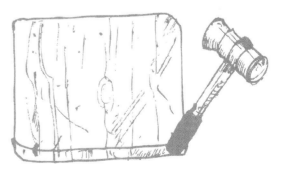

Pesto

There are endless variations on pesto – change out the basil for other herbs (mint is one of my favorites for roasted game or lamb) or even substitute spinach, kale or sundried tomatoes. Any nut can be used as well. This Paleo version omits the cheese in traditional recipes.

 Makes about 2 cups

- 2 cups packed fresh basil leaves
- ½ clove garlic
- ¼ cup pine nuts

- ⅔ cup extra virgin olive oil
- 1 tsp. lemon juice
- Freshly ground black pepper

•. Combine the basil, garlic, and pine nuts in a food processor and pulse until coarsely chopped. Add the oil and lemon juice and process until fully incorporated and smooth. Season with pepper.

Chef's Tip: This pumpkin seed variation is uniquely delicious. The recipe is included separately as the proportions are different than above.

- ½ cup plus 1 tbsp. extra virgin olive oil
- ¾ cup unsalted hulled green pumpkin seeds (also called pepitas)
- ¼ cup cilantro leaves

- 1 jalapeno pepper, seeded and stem removed
- 1 garlic clove, coarsely chopped
- 2 tbsps. lime juice
- Freshly ground black pepper to taste

1. In a large skillet, heat 1 tbsp. oil over medium heat. Add the pumpkin seeds and sauté, stirring constantly, until beginning to lightly brown and pop, about 2 minutes. Remove from heat and allow to cool.

2. In a food processor, combine the pumpkin seeds, cilantro, jalapeno and garlic, pulsing to chop. Add the lime juice and remaining olive oil and process until smooth. Add water a few teaspoons at a time and pulse until desired consistency is achieved.

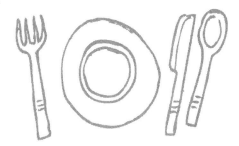

Tapenade

Tapenade is typically made with capers, which are not allowed on Paleo. This savory blend is still quite tasty and makes an excellent snack with the Lemon Pepper Crackers (see recipe p. 84) or some cut fresh vegetables for dipping. Add some to a simple chicken or fish dish for an extra layer of flavor.

 Makes 1 cup

- 3 tbsps. extra virgin olive oil
- 1 tbsp. lemon juice
- 1 tsp. minced garlic
- 2 anchovy fillets, in oil not salt, rinsed

- 1 tsp. chopped fresh basil
- 1 cup drained black olives, vinegar-free
- 1 tsp. freshly ground black pepper

- Blend the olive oil, lemon juice, garlic and anchovies together in a food processor until combined. Add basil and pulse to combine. Add olives and pepper and pulse until olives are in small pieces. Season with black pepper and refrigerate until serving.

Homemade Sausage

The seasonings may be varied according to when and how the sausage will be used. Add fresh sage for traditional breakfast sausage or minced garlic and fennel seeds for an Italian version.

 Makes 8 patties

- 1 tsp. chopped dried sage
- 1 tsp. chopped dried thyme
- ½ tsp. grated nutmeg
- ½ tsp. cayenne pepper
- ½ tsp. crushed red pepperflakes
- 1 tsp. freshly ground black pepper
- 1 lb. ground pork
- 2 tbsps. coconut oil

1. Combine sage, thyme, nutmeg, cayenne pepper, red pepper and black pepper in a large bowl. Add the pork and combine using a spoon or by hand.

2. If using for breakfast, add 1 tsp. fresh chopped sage. Divide the mixture evenly into 8 balls and flatten into patties. Heat the oil in a large non-stick skillet over medium heat. Add the patties and cook until lightly browned, about 4 minutes. Turn patties and cook until lightly browned and cooked through, about 3–4 minutes longer.

3. Sausage may be refrigerated uncooked for up to 2 days or frozen for up to 2 months.

Hollandaise

This Paleo version of hollandaise is made with olive oil instead of butter.

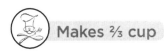 Makes ⅔ cup

- ½ cup dry white wine (or substitute 2 tbsps. lemon juice)
- 3 large egg yolks
- ½ cup extra virgin olive oil
- ½ tsp. white ground pepper
- ½ tsp. chopped chives

- Place white wine in the top of a double boiler and reduce by two-thirds. Whisk in the egg yolks and 2 tsps. warm water. Whisk the mixture until it's lemony and light, about 2–3 minutes. Remove from heat. Slowly whisk in olive oil, a little at a time. Continue whisking, adding remaining oil. Return to the heat briefly to reheat as necessary. Serve immediately.

Chef's Tip: Adding a little water to the egg yolks makes the texture fluffy and the mixture less likely to separate.

Tomato Salsa

Salsa is an all-purpose condiment that adds flavor to grilled chicken and fish. It's also a delicious snack when served with crackers.

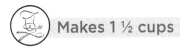 Makes 1 ½ cups

- 6 plum tomatoes, skins and seeds removed and coarsely chopped
- ½ red onion, coarsely chopped
- 8 scallions, trimmed and chopped
- 1 jalapeno pepper, seeded and finely chopped
- 3 tbsps. lime juice

- In a large bowl, mix together the tomatoes, red onions, half of the scallions and the jalapeno pepper. Mix in the lime juice and add fresh grated black pepper to taste. Refrigerate until ready to use. Garnish with remaining scallions to serve.

Chef's Tip: Hand chopping the tomatoes will result in a better texture than using a food processor, which can easily over-process them.

Mayonnaise

This mayonnaise has a richer flavor than standard mayo due to the addition of olive oil. Coconut oil is used to balance it out.

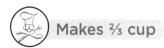 Makes ⅔ cup

- 1 egg yolk
- 1 tbsp. lemon juice

- ⅓ cup extra virgin olive oil
- ⅓ cup coconut oil, warmed to a liquid

- In a food processor or bowl, combine the egg yolk with the lemon juice and 2 tsps. warm water. With the food processor running (or whisking constantly), slowly drizzle the oil in a thin stream until mixture is smooth and thick. Cover and refrigerate for up to 4 days.

Chef's Tip: If you prefer to not use raw eggs, here is an easy method to pasteurize them:

- Place large egg(s) in a saucepan filled with water. Turn on the heat and bring the water up to 140 degrees F. using a digital thermometer for liquids clipped to the side of the pan. Maintain the water temperature at 140 degrees F. for 3 minutes (and no more than 142 degrees F.), adjusting the heat on the burner as necessary. Remove eggs from hot water and submerge in an ice water bath.

Salad Dressing

To make this salad dressing creamy, whisk in 1 egg with the lemon juice and shallot or 2 tbsps. of mayonnaise. Add seasonings and herbs to taste.

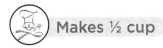 Makes ½ cup

- 3 tbsps. lemon or lime juice
- 2 tsps. chopped shallot

- ½ cup oil (olive, macadamia, avocado or walnut)

- Whisk together the lemon juice and shallot. With the food processor running (or whisking constantly), slowly drizzle in the oil until blended.

Chef's Tip: Prepare the dressing at least an hour ahead of serving and add desired herbs to allow the flavors to blend.

Chili Powder

Commercial chili powder often includes salt and sugar (among other things), so if a pure version is unavailable, it's best to make your own. It's simple and will last stored in an airtight container for a month.

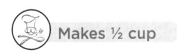 Makes ½ cup

- 1 cup dried chilies (ancho, chipotle, guajillo or mixed), seeds and stems removed

1. Preheat the oven to 300 degrees F. Line a baking sheet with parchment. Lay the chilies on the sheet in a single layer, and bake for 3–5 minutes until they are dry enough to crumble.

2. Remove from the oven and cool slightly. Crumble the chilies into a small bowl. Transfer to a spice grinder or food processor and grind to a powder. Store in an airtight container for up to 1 month.

Chapter 4

Breakfasts

- Almond Crusted Crab Cakes with Poached Eggs
- Breakfast Wraps with Chorizo, Eggs and Salsa
- Salmon Frittata
- Blueberry Pancakes with Peaches
- Pumpkin and Apple Pancakes
- Steak and Egg Custards
- Wilted Spinach and Crab in Egg Crepes
- Portobello Mushrooms with Eggs and Basil

- Oven Puffed Lobster Custards
- Baked Eggs with Pork and Mushrooms
- Caramelized Onion Omelet
- Scrambled Eggs with Eggplant
- Middle Eastern Eggs
- Cinnamon Crepes with Berries
- Avocado Eggs Benedict
- Duck and Egg Casserole

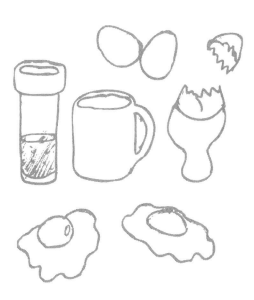

Almond Crusted Crab Cakes with Poached Eggs

This dish is elegant for brunch but equally at home on the dinner table.

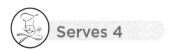 **Serves 4**

- 6 tbsps. mayonnaise (see recipe p. 54)
- ¼ teaspoon paprika
- ⅛ teaspoon cayenne pepper
- ⅛ tsp. ground dry mustard
- ⅛ tsp. ground allspice

- 2 tsps. chopped fresh flat-leaf parsley
- 2 tbsps. almond flour
- 9 large eggs
- 1 lb. fresh lump crabmeat
- 1 tsp. paprika
- ½ cup sliced almonds

1. Preheat the oven to 350 degrees F. Line a baking sheet with parchment and set aside.

2. In a medium bowl, combine 3 tbsps. mayonnaise with the paprika, cayenne pepper, mustard and allspice. Stir in the parsley and almond flour. Whisk 1 egg in a small bowl or measuring cup. Stir the egg into the mixture. Gently fold the crabmeat into the mayonnaise mixture. Divide the mixture into 8 parts and shape into crab cakes. Place crab cakes onto the baking sheet and sprinkle with paprika.

3. Bake the crab cakes for 15 minutes. Remove from the oven and spoon the remaining mayonnaise evenly over the crab cakes. Divide the almonds evenly over the crab cakes and return to the oven. Bake 4–5 minutes longer, until lightly browned.

4 Poach the eggs while the crab cakes finish baking (see Technique p. 34). Place poached eggs onto crab cakes to serve.

Chef's Note: The combination of paprika, cayenne pepper, ground mustard and allspice makes a tasty all-purpose seafood rub.

Breakfast Wraps with Chorizo, Eggs and Salsa

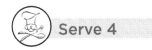 Serve 4

Napa cabbage makes a delicious alternative wrap to tortillas or even lettuce leaves. Fresh chorizo is a blend of ground pork with specific spices and seasonings. If you prefer to use less pork, store any leftovers in the freezer for an easy meal. It's delicious baked in bell peppers.

- 8 large eggs
- 2 tbsps. crushed red pepperflakes
- 1 tsp. minced garlic
- ½ tsp. ground coriander
- ½ tsp. ground cumin
- 2 tsps. smoked paprika
- 1 ½ tsps. chopped oregano
- 1 lb. ground pork

- 3 tbsps. extra virgin olive oil
- 6 scallions, ends trimmed and coarsely chopped
- ½ cup sliced mushrooms
- Freshly ground pepper to taste
- 1 avocado, peeled, seeded and sliced
- 1 cup fresh Tomato Salsa (see recipe p. 53)

1. In a large bowl, whisk the eggs and set aside.

2. Make the chorizo. In a food processor, add the red pepper flakes, minced garlic, coriander, cumin, paprika and oregano and pulse until combined. Pulse until all the spices are evenly mixed. Place the pork into a large bowl. Sprinkle the seasoning over it and mix to combine.

3. In a large skillet, heat 1 tbsp. olive oil over medium heat. Crumble in the sausage and sauté until it begins to brown, about 3–4 minutes. Remove from pan and drain any excess fat. Return the pan to the heat and add 1 tbsp. olive oil. Stir in the remaining scallions and mushrooms and cook until soft, about 4–5 minutes. Stir in the scrambled eggs and lower the heat. Cook until eggs are soft and glossy. Stir the sausage back into the eggs and remove from heat.

4. Lay out 8 Napa cabbage leaves and divide the filling among them. Divide the avocado pieces between them. Season with freshly ground black pepper. Serve with the fresh salsa.

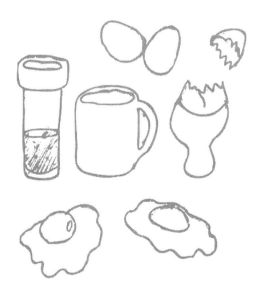

Salmon Frittata

This is a delicious way to incorporate omega-3 rich salmon into breakfast. Poach, grill or panfry an extra piece when making lunch or dinner and have it ready for this savory frittata.

 Serves 4

- 8 large eggs
- 3 tbsps. coconut oil
- 1 shallot, peeled and finely chopped
- 1 cup peeled and grated sweet potato

- 8- to 10-oz. salmon filet, fully cooked, skin removed and crumbled into chunks
- 2 tsps. chopped fresh dill
- Freshly ground pepper to taste

1. Preheat the broiler on low. In a large bowl, whisk the eggs and set aside.

2. In a large oven-proof skillet, heat the oil over medium heat. Add the shallot and cook for 1 minute. Add the shredded sweet potato and cook for 5–7 minutes, until tender but not brown. Add the salmon and stir until just heated through. Pour the eggs over the potato salmon mixture. Stir until just combined. Lower the heat and cook until the edges start to brown and the eggs are set but still loose in the center, about 6–8 minutes. Place the pan under the broiler and continue cooking until eggs are firm and cooked through, about 3–4 minutes. Sprinkle on the fresh dill and season with pepper. Cut into wedges to serve.

Blueberry Pancakes with Peaches

Wild Maine blueberries are sweeter and more flavorful than most farmed berries. If you can find them in the frozen food section, they are a delicious addition to these pancakes (if local berries are unavailable).

 Makes 8–10 pancakes

- 3 large eggs, separated
- ¼ cup coconut milk
- 1 tbsp. vanilla extract
- 1 ½ cups almond flour
- 1 tsp. ground cinnamon
- 1 tsp. baking soda

- 1 cup blueberries
- ¼ cup coconut cream, whipped to soft peaks
- 2 large ripe peaches, skin and stones removed, cut into thin slices

1. Beat the egg whites until soft peaks form, then set aside. In a large bowl, whisk together the eggs yolks, coconut milk and vanilla. In a separate large bowl, combine the almond flour, cinnamon and baking powder. Fold the egg yolk mixture into the dry ingredients until just combined. Add water a teaspoon at a time as necessary (until the batter drips off the spatula). Fold the egg whites into the batter until just incorporated. Gently fold in the blueberries.

2. Heat a large nonstick skillet over medium high heat. When skillet is hot enough for a drop of water to sizzle, lower the heat and spoon about 2–3 tbsps. of the batter onto the skillet, forming a pancake about 3 inches in diameter. Spread the batter to form a uniform circle. Repeat, leaving space between the pancakes. Cook until dry around the edges and bubbles have formed over the top, about 2–3 minutes. Flip and continue cooking until done in the middle and golden brown, about 2–3 minutes more.

3. Serve with coconut cream and peaches.

Pumpkin and Apple Pancakes

These pancakes take longer to cook than standard wheat flour pancakes so keep the heat low to avoid burning them.

 Makes 8–10 pancakes

- 5 large eggs, separated
- ¾ cup coconut milk
- ½ cup pumpkin puree
- 2 tsps. vanilla extract
- ¼ cup coconut flour
- 1 cup almond flour
- 1 tsp. baking soda
- ½ tsp. ground ginger
- ½ tsp. ground nutmeg
- ¼ tsp. ground clove
- 1 cup finely chopped apples
- 2 tbsps. coconut oil
- ¼ cup coconut cream, whipped to soft peaks

1. In a large bowl, whisk the egg whites to soft peaks (or use an electric mixer). In a separate bowl, whisk together the egg yolks and coconut milk. Add the pumpkin and vanilla and whisk to combine. In a separate large bowl, combine the coconut and almond flours, baking soda, ginger, nutmeg and clove. Fold the egg yolk mixture into the dry ingredients until just combined. Add water a teaspoon at a time as necessary (until the batter drips off the spatula). Gently fold in the egg whites until just combined. Fold the apples into the batter.

2. Heat a large nonstick skillet over low heat. Brush lightly with coconut oil. When skillet is hot enough for a drop of water to sizzle, lower the heat and spoon about 2–3 tbsps. of the batter onto the skillet, forming a pancake about 3 inches in diameter. Spread the batter to form a uniform circle. Repeat, leaving space between pancakes. Cook until dry around the edges and bubbles have formed on the top, about 5 minutes. Flip and continue cooking until done in the middle and golden brown, about 5 minutes more.

3. Serve with coconut cream.

Steak and Egg Custards

Cooking these delicious custards in a warm water bath creates their creamy texture.

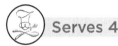 **Serves 4**

- 2–3 tbsps. extra virgin olive oil
- ¼ chopped onion
- 1 (8-oz) boneless steak, chopped into ½-inch chunks
- 1 cup coconut milk

- 8 large eggs
- ¼ tsp. cayenne pepper
- Freshly ground black pepper to taste
- 1 tsp. chopped fresh thyme

1. Preheat the oven to 350 degrees F. Brush the insides of 4 individual ramekins with 1–2 tbsps. oil and set aside.

2. Heat the remaining 1 tbsp. oil in a medium skillet over medium heat. Add the onion and cook until just softened, about 3–4 minutes. Add the steak and cook until lightly browned, stirring constantly, about 2 minutes. Divide the mixture evenly among the ramekins.

3. Heat the coconut milk in a small saucepan over medium heat until steaming. Whisk the eggs in a large bowl. Slowly pour the coconut milk mixture over them, whisking continuously until well combined. Stir in the cayenne pepper. Divide the mixture evenly among the ramekins.

4. Place ramekins into a roasting pan. Fill the pan with very hot water halfway up the sides of the cups. Bake 20–25 minutes until lightly browned and just cooked through. Remove from the water bath and allow to cool slightly. Season with black pepper and sprinkle on the thyme to serve.

Chef's Note: Substitute different game meats like venison or elk for an interesting variation.

Wilted Spinach and Crab in Egg Crepes

Spinach combines with crab for an elegant yet healthy breakfast treat.

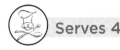 Serves 4

- 2 cups baby spinach, stems removed
- 6 large eggs
- ½ tsp. finely ground white or black pepper
- ¼ tsp. cayenne pepper
- 2 tbsps. chopped chives

- 2 tbsps. coconut oil
- 1 tsp. chopped shallot
- ½ lb. fresh lump crabmeat
- ¼ cup coconut cream
- Pinch of nutmeg
- 2 tsps. chopped flat-leaf parsley

1. Preheat the oven to 350 degrees F. Line a baking sheet with parchment and set aside. Blanch the baby spinach for 30 seconds until wilted. Cool in ice bath, then roll in paper towels to dry. Set aside.

2. Whisk the eggs, cayenne pepper and chives together in a small bowl. Heat 1 tbsp. coconut oil in a medium skillet over medium heat. Pour in about 1/4 cup of the eggs and quickly swirl to evenly coat the entire bottom. Cook until set but not brown, about 30 seconds. Carefully flip and cook on the other side until just cooked through, about 15–20 seconds longer. Transfer the egg crepe to a plate and repeat process until all batter is used (you will have 4–6 crepes when finished).

3. In a small skillet, melt the remaining 1 tbsp. coconut oil over medium heat. Stir in the shallot and cook until just softened, about 30 seconds. Add the crabmeat and stir until just heated through. Add the coconut cream and cook until mixture is just thickened. Stir in the spinach and cook until heated through. Remove from heat and stir in the nutmeg. Allow to cool and thicken slightly, about 4–5 minutes.

4. Divide the spinach crab mixture among the crepes. Roll up and place each crepe on the prepared pan. Cover with aluminum foil. When ready to serve, place the covered crepes into the oven and heat for 4–6 minutes, until just heated through. Sprinkle with parsley to serve.

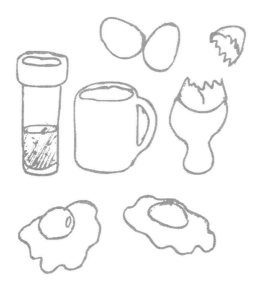

Portobello Mushrooms with Eggs and Basil

Portobello mushrooms have a meaty texture that stands up well to broiling and grilling.

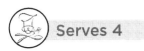 **Serves 4**

- 1 tsp. minced garlic
- 4 tbsps. extra virgin olive oil
- 4 large Portobello caps, gills removed if desired (see Tip below)
- Freshly ground black pepper

- 6 large eggs
- 2 tbsps. coconut milk
- ¼ cup fresh chopped basil
- 3 plum tomatoes, seeded and coarsely chopped

1. Heat the broiler on high.

2. In a small bowl or measuring cup, whisk together the garlic and 3 tbsps. olive oil. Brush the mushrooms with garlic oil on both sides. Place onto a baking sheet with undersides up and season with black pepper. Place under the broiler and cook for 3 minutes. Turn the mushrooms and cook 3–4 minutes longer, until tender. Remove from the broiler and keep warm. (Alternately cook them on a preheated grill for the same amount of time).

3. Heat the remaining 1 tbsp. olive oil in a small nonstick saucepan or skillet over medium heat. Break the eggs into the pan and lower the heat. Stir eggs to combine. When eggs just begin to clump, stir in the coconut milk. Continue to stir gently until eggs are cooked but still glossy. Remove from heat and stir in the basil.

4. Place the mushrooms on a plate with their undersides up. Divide the eggs evenly among the mushrooms. Top the eggs with the chopped tomato to serve.

Chef's Tip: The dark gills found on the underside of a Portobello are edible but can turn your filling black and unappetizing. If presentation matters, scrape them off with a spoon or paring knife.

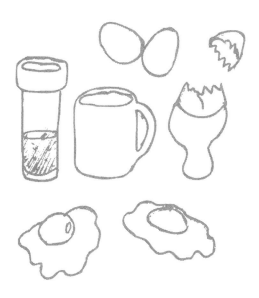

Oven Puffed Lobster Custards

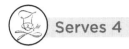 Serves 4

- 1 tbsp. coconut oil
- 6 large eggs
- ¾ cup coconut milk
- 2 tsps. chopped dill

- 1 cup fresh Maine lobster meat, coarsely chopped
- 2 scallions, ends trimmed and coarsely chopped

1. Preheat the oven to 400 degrees F. Lightly grease 4 custard cups or individual ramekins with the coconut oil.

2. In a large bowl, whisk together the eggs and the coconut milk. Stir in the dill. Fill each cup about half full of the egg mixture. Divide the lobster and scallions evenly among the cups. Top each with the remaining egg mixture. Bake until puffed and beginning to brown, about 15–20 minutes. Serve immediately.

Baked Eggs with Pork and Mushrooms

Baked eggs are simple and delicious. Keep a close eye on them towards the end of the baking to make sure they do not overcook.

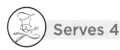 **Serves 4**

- 2 tbsps. coconut oil
- 1 tbsp. extra virgin olive oil
- 1 shallot, peeled and finely chopped
- 1 cup mushrooms, finely chopped
- ¼ lb. ground pork
- 1 tsp. chopped fresh thyme
- 4 large eggs
- Freshly ground pepper to taste
- 4 tsps. coconut cream, warmed to a liquid
- 2 tbsps. chopped fresh flat leaf parsley

1. Preheat an oven to 350 degrees F. Brush the coconut oil liberally into 4 individual 5- to 6-oz. ramekins.

2. Heat the olive oil in a medium skillet over medium high heat. Add the shallots and cook for 30 seconds. Add the mushrooms and cook for 1 minute, stirring constantly. Add the ground pork and cook for 3–4 minutes, until just cooked through. Remove from heat and stir in the thyme.

3. Divide the mixture among the prepared ramekins. Break an egg into each ramekin. Season the eggs with black pepper. Drizzle the top of each egg with 1 tsp. of the cream. Arrange the ramekins on a rimmed baking sheet. Bake until the egg whites are opaque and the yolks have firm edges and are soft in the center, about 12–15 minutes. Remove from the oven and sprinkle each egg evenly with parsley.

Chef's Tip: Substitute ground turkey for pork if desired.

Caramelized Onion Omelet

Caramelizing onions brings out their sweetness and adds a nutty flavor.

 Serves 4

- 2–3 tbsps. extra virgin olive oil
- 1 ½ cups sliced sweet onion
- 1 clove garlic, minced
- 8 large eggs

- ½ tsp. cayenne pepper
- Pinch of nutmeg (optional)
- Freshly ground pepper to taste

1. Heat 1 tbsp. oil over medium heat in a medium skillet. Add the onion, lower heat and cook, stirring often, until onion is softened and caramelized, about 15–18 minutes. Add the garlic and stir for 30 seconds. Remove from heat and set aside to cool slightly.

2. In a medium bowl, whisk together the eggs, pepper and nutmeg.

3. Heat a medium nonstick skillet over medium heat. Brush the pan with olive oil. Pour 1/4 of the egg mixture into the center of the pan and tilt the pan to spread the egg mixture evenly. Let eggs firm up a little, and after about 10 seconds shake the pan a bit and use a spatula to gently direct the mixture away from the sides and into the middle. Allow any liquid to flow to the sides. Cook for 2–3 minutes until the egg mixture holds together. Spoon 1/4 of the onions into the center. Use a spatula to fold the omelet over into half or thirds. Keep warm.

4. Repeat with the remaining eggs until 4 omelets are complete. Season with black pepper.

Chef's Tip: Caramelized onions are delicious any time of day served over grilled or roasted meats.

Scrambled Eggs with Eggplant

The addition of eggplant and turmeric lends an exotic taste to this delicious scrambled egg dish.

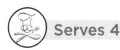 **Serves 4**

- 3 tbsps. extra virgin olive oil
- 4 Japanese eggplants, tops trimmed and cut in half
- 6 large tomatoes, chopped
- 2 tsps. minced garlic

- 2 tsps. turmeric
- 8 large eggs, lightly whisked
- 1 large cucumber, peeled, seeded and cut into ½-inch dice
- 1 tsp. chopped mint

1. Preheat the oven to 375 degrees F. Lightly grease an 8" x 8" baking dish with 1 tbsp. olive oil and set aside.

2. Prick the eggplants all over and place on a baking sheet cut side up. Bake for about 18–20 minutes or until very tender. Coarsely chop the eggplant and spoon into a medium bowl. Stir in the tomatoes.

3. Heat the oil in a medium skillet over medium high heat. Add the garlic and cook for 30 seconds. Add the turmeric and cook for 30 seconds longer. Pour in the eggs and stir to scramble. Stir until the eggs are cooked through but still glossy. Stir in the eggplant mixture and cook until just heated through. Sprinkle on the cucumber and mint to serve.

Middle Eastern Eggs

This traditional Middle Eastern dish (sometimes called "Shakshuka," meaning "a mixture") is made Paleo friendly by eliminating cheese and the toast traditionally served with it.

 Serves 4

- ¼ cup extra virgin olive oil
- 2 jalapeno peppers, stemmed, seeded and finely chopped
- 1 small yellow onion, chopped
- 2 tsps. minced garlic
- 1 tsp. ground cumin
- ½ tsp. turmeric
- 1 tbsp. paprika
- 1 (28-oz.) can crushed or diced tomatoes
- Freshly ground black pepper to taste
- 8 large eggs
- 1 tbsp. chopped mint

1. Heat oil in a large skillet over medium-high heat. Add the jalapenos and onions and cook, stirring occasionally, until soft and golden brown, about 4–5 minutes. Add garlic, cumin, turmeric and paprika, and cook, stirring frequently, until garlic is soft, about 1 minute longer.

2. Add the tomatoes and their liquid to the skillet. Stir in 1/2 cup water, reduce heat to medium and simmer until thickened slightly, about 20 minutes. Season with pepper.

3. Remove the pan from the heat. Make 8 indentations to accommodate the eggs evenly distributed around the pan. Crack the eggs into the indentations in the sauce. Return the pan to the heat and cook for about 10 minutes, basting the eggs occasionally to cook evenly. Cover the skillet and cook until yolks are just set, about 2–3 minutes longer (add 3–4 minutes for well done). Sprinkle with mint to serve.

Cinnamon Crepes with Berries

Easy to make ahead, crepes are always a sophisticated addition to any breakfast menu.

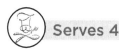 **Serves 4**

- 4 eggs
- ⅓ cup almond flour
- 1 teaspoon vanilla extract
- ¼ tsp. cinnamon
- 3 tbsps. coconut oil
- 1 cup blueberries
- 1 tsp. lemon juice
- 1 pint strawberries, sliced

1. In a medium bowl, whisk the eggs. Stir in the almond flour and vanilla. Add water a teaspoon at a time as necessary to form a thin batter. Allow the batter to rest for 15 minutes.

2. Brush a medium skillet with coconut oil and heat over medium heat. Pour 1/4 cup of the batter into the pan. Swirl the pan immediately so that the batter coats the entire base of the pan. Cook for 1–2 minutes until the edge begins to brown and curl. Turn the crepe and cook for 20 seconds longer. Remove from the pan. Repeat to form seven more crepes.

3. Heat 1 tbsp. coconut oil in a small saucepan on medium heat. Add the blueberries. Stir in the lemon juice. Allow the mixture to begin to bubble, then reduce heat to low. Cook, stirring often, until the berries pop and release their juices. Add the strawberries and cook for 1 minute longer.

4. To serve, fill crepes with berries or fold crepes into quarters and spoon berries on top.

Chef's Tip: If making crepes ahead, layer them with parchment and store in a Ziploc bag in the refrigerator for up to 3 days. Remove parchment and reheat at 350 degrees F. for about 1–2 minutes before serving. The sweetness of this dish depends on the fruit, so choose only the ripest berries.

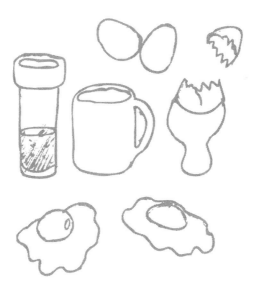

Avocado Eggs Benedict

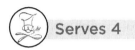 Serves 4

- 3 large ripe avocados, peeled, seeded and diced
- 2 tsps. lime juice
- 3 plum tomatoes, seeded and diced
- 1 jalapeno pepper, seeded and minced
- 1 tbsp. chopped cilantro
- 8 large eggs
- Freshly ground black pepper to taste
- ⅔ cup Hollandaise sauce (see recipe p. 52)

1. Place the chopped avocado into a medium bowl. Toss avocado with lime juice. Stir in the tomatoes, pepper and cilantro.

2. Divide the avocado mixture between 4 plates. Poach the eggs (see Technique p. 34) and spoon them onto the avocado. Season with pepper to taste. Divide the hollandaise sauce evenly among the eggs to serve.

Duck and Egg Casserole

Muscovy duck breast without the skin is actually lower in saturated fat than chicken. Duck adds a rich flavor to this simple breakfast casserole.

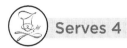 **Serves 4**

- 3 tbsps. olive oil
- 2 shallots, peeled and finely chopped
- 4 sweet potatoes, peeled and grated
- ½ tsp. chopped thyme

- 1 cup chopped duck breast (or other cooked meat)
- 6 large eggs
- ⅓ cup coconut milk
- ¼ tsp. cayenne pepper
- 2 tbsps. chopped flat-leaf parsley
- Freshly ground pepper to taste

1. Preheat the oven to 350 degrees F. Lightly grease an 8" x 8" baking dish with 1 tbsp. olive oil and set aside.

2. Heat the remaining 2 tbsps. olive oil in a large skillet over medium-high heat. Add the shallot and cook, stirring constantly, for 2 minutes. Add the sweet potatoes and cook 4–5 minutes, until they begin to soften. Stir in the thyme and remove from heat.

3. Spread the potato mixture evenly in the bottom of the baking dish. Layer on the duck meat. In a medium bowl, whisk together the eggs, coconut milk, cayenne pepper and parsley. Pour the mixture over the duck and potatoes. Bake for 25–30 minutes, until eggs are firm and cooked through. Season with freshly ground pepper. Allow to cool slightly before cutting into squares to serve.

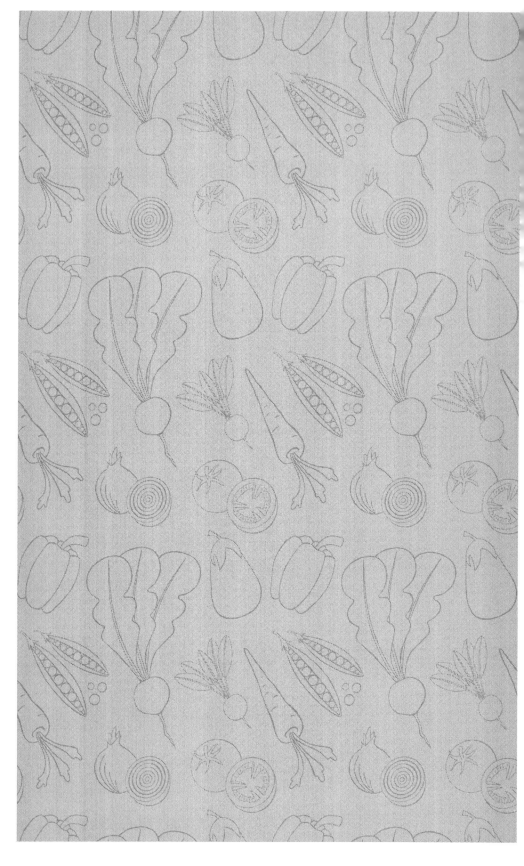

Chapter 5

Snacks and Starters

- Roasted Eggplant Dip
- Marcona Almonds with Rosemary and Olives
- Pumpkin Seed Hummus
- Oysters with Spinach and Coconut Milk
- Lemon Pepper Crackers
- Parsnip and Beet Chips
- Spiced Nuts
- Chicken Liver Pate
- Chilled Mussels with Tomatoes, Onions and Basil
- Ceviche with Avocado and Watermelon
- Shrimp with Fennel Seeds and Lemon
- Chicken Satay with Cashews
- Beef Skewers with Mustard and Scallions
- Green Vegetable Dip

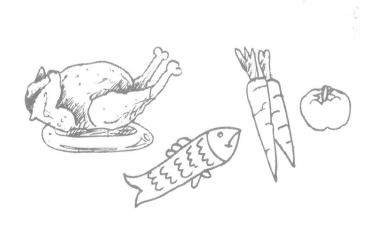

Roasted Eggplant Dip

Tahini, or sesame paste, adds a Middle Eastern flavor to this easy-to-prepare dip. Serve with raw vegetables for dipping for a tasty snack.

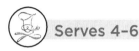 **Serves 4–6**

- 1 large eggplant
- ¼ cup tahini
- I tsp. minced garlic
- ½ tsp. cayenne pepper

- ¼ cup lemon juice
- 2 tbsps. extra virgin olive oil
- 1 tbsp. chopped Italian parsley
- Freshly ground black pepper to taste

- Preheat the oven to 375 degrees F. Prick the skin of the eggplant a few times. Place the eggplant onto a baking sheet and roast in the oven for 20–30 minutes, until completely soft. Remove from the oven and allow to cool. Split the eggplant in half and scrape out the pulp into the bowl of a food processor. Add the tahini and process until smooth. Add the garlic, cayenne pepper, lemon juice and olive oil and combine until smooth. Add the parsley and pulse just to combine. Season with black pepper to taste.

Marcona Almonds with Rosemary and Olives

This pan roasted combination of almonds and olives makes a tasty snack.

 Makes 1 ½ cups

- 2 tbsps. extra virgin olive oil
- 1 cup whole blanched Marcona almonds
- ½ cup drained black olives
- 2 tsps. fresh chopped rosemary

- Heat the olive oil in a large skillet over medium heat. Add the almonds and toss to coat. Cook the almonds for 2–3 minutes, until lightly browned. Add the olives and stir to coat and just heat through, about 1 minute longer. Remove from the heat and stir in the rosemary. Allow to cool slightly but serve warm.

Pumpkin Seed Hummus

This savory Paleo friendly blend of pumpkin seeds and sesame paste has the texture of traditional hummus.

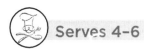 **Serves 4-6**

- 2 cups unsalted hulled green pumpkin seeds (also called pepitas)
- 1 tsp. minced garlic
- 1 ½ tsps. smoked paprika
- ½ tsp. cayenne pepper

- ½ cup plus 1 tbsp. olive oil
- ¼ cup tahini
- 3 tbsps. lemon juice
- Freshly ground pepper to taste
- ½ cup chopped scallions for garnish

1. Preheat oven to 325 degrees F. Line a baking sheet with parchment or aluminum foil.

2. In a medium bowl, mix together the pumpkin seeds, garlic, smoked paprika, cayenne pepper and 1 tbsp. of olive oil. Spread the seeds out onto the baking sheet. Roast for 12–15 minutes until seeds are cooked and toasted a light brown. Remove from the oven and allow seeds to cool.

3. Add the pumpkin seeds to a food processor and process until a smooth paste forms, scraping down the sides as needed. Add the tahini and process until combined. With the food processor turned on, drizzle in the remaining 1/2 cup of olive oil and blend continuously until smooth. Add the lemon juice and pulse just until combined. Season with black pepper and garnish with scallions to serve.

Oysters with Spinach and Coconut Milk

Coconut milk is infused with lemongrass in this Paleo friendly version of oysters Florentine.

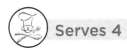 Serves 4

- 1 stalk lemongrass
- ⅓ cup coconut milk
- 1 tsp. lemon juice
- 2 tbsps. coconut oil
- 1 garlic clove, minced
- 1 shallot, chopped
- 2 cups fresh baby spinach
- 20 fresh oysters on the half shell
- Rock salt for baking (optional)

1. Cut the top off the stalk of lemongrass, about 6 inches from the bottom. Crush the lemongrass with the back of a knife to break it up and then chop it into coarse pieces. In a small saucepan, bring the coconut milk and lemongrass pieces to a boil. Simmer over low heat for 5 minutes to infuse and thicken. Let cool. Strain out the lemongrass and discard, reserving the coconut milk. Stir in the lemon juice and set aside.

2. Heat the oil in a large skillet over medium heat. Add the garlic and shallot and sauté for 1 minute. Add the spinach and cook for 1–2 minutes until the spinach just wilts. Pour in the coconut milk and cook until just beginning to bubble and thicken, about 2 minutes. Spoon 1 heaping teaspoon of the spinach mixture onto each oyster. Sprinkle a baking pan with rock salt to hold oysters. Arrange the oysters in the salt. Bake for 8–10 minutes until hot and just cooked through.

Chef's Tip: Rock salt creates a stable base on which to bake the oysters and retains heat for serving.

Lemon Pepper Crackers

These crackers are tasty on their own and excellent served with the recipes for dips. The seasoning is adjusted to not compete with dips or salsas. Include herbs like rosemary or seasonings like paprika to add flavor. The cayenne pepper adds a little kick but can be omitted if a less peppery taste is desired.

 Makes 40-50 crackers

- 2 cups almond flour
- 1 tbsp. lemon zest
- ¼ tsp. cayenne pepper
- 1 tsp. coarsely ground black pepper

- 1 large egg
- 2 tsps. lemon juice
- 4 tsps. extra virgin olive oil

1. Preheat the oven to 350 degrees. Line two 12" x 16" baking sheets with parchment and set aside.

2. In a large bowl, combine almond flour, lemon zest, cayenne pepper and 3/4 tsp. black pepper.

3. In a separate bowl or measuring cup, whisk together the egg, lemon juice and olive oil. Pour the wet ingredients into the dry ingredients and mix with a pastry blender or a fork until combined. Divide the dough in half.

4. Form half of the mixture by hand into a log about 3–4 inches long. Place the log onto 1 of the baking sheets lined with parchment. Top with a second piece of parchment paper. Press the dough lengthwise on the pan into an oval shape about 6" x 8" (the goal is to get as close to a rectangle as possible). Use a rolling pin to roll the dough thinly and evenly. Remove the top layer of parchment. Trim the edges of the dough into a rectangle using a sharp knife.

Put the scraps with the remaining half of dough. Cut the dough into 1 1/2" strips and then approximately 1 1/2" squares. Use the knife to separate the squares at least 1" apart so the edges will brown evenly. Prick each square twice with a fork. Sprinkle the remaining 1/4 tsp. black pepper evenly over top.

5. Bake at 350 degrees F. for 8–10 minutes or until golden brown around the edges. Watch carefully the last few minutes as the thinner the crackers are, the more quickly they will brown. Place on a cooling rack. When cool, store in an airtight container. Repeat with remaining dough, incorporating the scraps.

Chef's Tip: The crackers may also be cut out into rounds with a small-diameter cookie cutter.

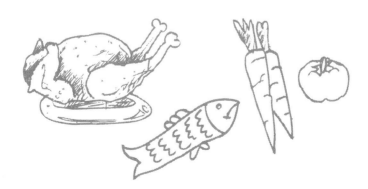

Parsnip and Beet Chips

Thinly sliced root vegetables bake into a crispy and easily prepared treat.

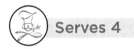 **Serves 4**

- 3 medium parsnips, peeled and ends trimmed
- 3 medium beets, peeled
- 2 tbsps. extra virgin olive oil
- 1 tsp. smoked paprika
- 1 tsp. Chili Powder (see recipe p. 56)
- Freshly ground pepper to taste

1. Preheat oven to 350 degrees F. Line two baking sheets with parchment and set aside.

2. Cut the parsnips into paper-thin coin shaped slices. Place the sliced parsnips onto a paper towel in a single layer for about 10 minutes to remove excess moisture. Similarly, slice the beets into coins and lay them out on paper towels to dry slightly. Add the parsnip and beet chips to a large bowl and toss with the oil. Sprinkle with paprika and chili powder and toss to coat evenly.

3. Place chips onto the baking sheets in a single layer. Bake for 20 minutes. Flip the chips over and bake for 10–15 minutes longer, until lightly browned. Transfer the chips to a cooling rack or paper towels and allow to cool and crisp.

Spiced Nuts

These are easy to make and turn out perfectly every time. Substitute curry powder or other seasonings to create different flavors.

 Makes 4 cups

- 4 tbsps. lime juice
- 1 tbsp. cayenne pepper
- 1 tbsp. smoked paprika or chili powder

- 4 cups unsalted mixed nuts, such as walnuts, pecans, hazelnuts and almonds

- Preheat the oven to 250 degrees F. In a large bowl, whisk together the lime juice and seasonings. Add nuts and toss to coat. Divide the nuts between 2 large rimmed baking sheets. Spread nuts evenly and place in the oven for 15 minutes. Stir the nuts then return to the oven for 15 minutes. Stir again and then cook 10–15 minutes longer, until nuts are dry. Let cool completely. Store in an airtight container.

Chicken Liver Pate

Creamy chicken liver pate stuffed in celery makes a delicious hors d'ouevres.

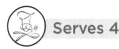 Serves 4

- 2 tbsps. coconut oil (or use rendered chicken fat)
- 1 cup chopped yellow onions
- 1 lb. chicken livers
- 1 bay leaf
- ½ tsp. ground allspice
- 1 tsp. chopped fresh thyme

- ½ teaspoon freshly ground black pepper
- ¼ cup Madeira (optional)
- 2 hardboiled eggs, coarsely chopped
- Chopped parsley leaves, for garnish

1. In a large sauté pan or skillet, heat 2 tbsps. coconut oil over medium-high heat. Add the onions and cook, stirring, until soft, about 3 minutes. Add the chicken livers, bay leaf, allspice, thyme and pepper. Cook, stirring constantly, until the livers are browned on the outside and still slightly pink on the inside, about 5 minutes. Add the Madeira if using and cook until most of the liquid is evaporated and the livers are cooked through but still tender.

2. Remove from the heat and let cool slightly. Discard the bay leaves.

3. In a food processor, puree the liver mixture. Add the eggs and process until smooth. Press the mixture through a mesh sieve before chilling,

4. Pack the pate into ramekins or jars. Garnish with parsley if desired. Cover with plastic and refrigerate until firm, at least 6 hours.

Chilled Mussels with Tomatoes, Onions and Basil

Sometimes the simplest dishes can be the most satisfying when using fresh ingredients.

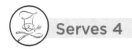 **Serves 4**

- ½ cup white wine (optional)
- 2 lbs. small mussels, scrubbed and de-bearded
- 4 plum tomatoes, seeded and coarsely chopped
- ½ cup chopped onion
- 3 tbsps. chopped fresh basil
- 2 tbsps. lemon juice

1. Pour the wine into a stockpot if using. Add 1 cup water to stockpot and bring to a boil over high heat. Add the mussels and cover. Bring back to a boil and cook for 4–5 minutes. Remove any opened mussels and set aside. Continue cooking 3 minutes longer. Remove any opened mussels and discard any unopened ones. Allow to cool. Remove mussels from shells, reserving half the shells. Allow the mussels to cool. Refrigerate to chill through, at least 30 minutes.

2. In a medium bowl, combine the tomatoes, onion, basil and lemon juice. Spread the mussel shells out on a platter and place a chilled mussel in each shell. Divide the tomato mixture evenly among the mussels. Cover and refrigerate for at least 30 minutes before serving.

Chef's Tip: Mussels can be prepared up to 8 hours ahead and refrigerated until ready to serve.

Ceviche with Avocado and Watermelon

Lime juice cooks the fish in this lively combination of fresh flavors and textures.

 Serves 4

- 1 lb. fresh, skinless snapper, sea bass or halibut, cut into 1/2-inch dice
- 1 ½ cups fresh lime juice
- ¼ cup coarsely chopped red onion
- 3 plum tomatoes, seeded and diced
- 2 jalapeno peppers, stemmed, seeded and finely chopped

- ⅓ cup chopped cilantro
- 3 tbsps. avocado oil
- Freshly ground pepper to taste
- 1 large ripe avocado
- 1 cup diced watermelon
- 2 tsps. black sesame seeds (optional)

1. In a large glass bowl, combine the fish, lime juice and onion. Use enough juice to cover the fish and allow it to float freely. Cover and refrigerate for about 4 hours, until a cube of fish no longer looks raw when broken open. Drain in a colander and discard juice.

2. In a large bowl, mix together the tomatoes, peppers, cilantro and oil. Stir in the fish and season with pepper. Cover and refrigerate if not serving immediately. Just before serving, peel, pit and dice the avocado and fold into mixture. Fold in the watermelon to serve. Toss mixture with sesame seeds if using to serve.

Shrimp with Fennel Seeds and Lemon

Fennel seeds provide a tasty variation to a Paleo version of shrimp scampi.

 Serves 4

- 2 tbsps. coconut oil
- 1 lb. extra-large shrimp, peeled and deveined but tails left on (about 20 shrimp)

- 1 tsp. minced garlic
- 1 tsp. whole fennel seeds
- 2 tbsps. lemon juice

- Heat the coconut oil in a large skillet over medium-high heat. Add the shrimp and cook until edges begin to brown, about 3–4 minutes. Turn shrimp over and cook until opaque, about 1–2 minutes longer. Add the garlic and cook for 30 seconds. Add the fennel seeds and stir to combine. Remove from the heat and stir in the lemon juice. Serve warm.

Chicken Satay with Cashews

Cashews are ground with coconut milk and spices to add a distinct flavor to this savory satay.

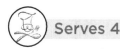 **Serves 4**

- 2 (6- to 8-oz.) boneless skinless chicken breasts
- 1 cup coconut milk
- 2–4 tbsps. lime juice
- 2 cloves garlic, crushed

- 1 tbsp. minced fresh ginger
- 1 Thai chili pepper, seeded and minced
- 1 cup cashews

1. Slice each piece of chicken into 6–8 long strips approximately a half inch thick. Pound out the chicken slightly to flatten it to an even thickness. In a shallow bowl, whisk together 1/2 cup coconut milk, 1 tbsp. lime juice, garlic and ginger. Add the chicken strips to the mixture and toss to coat. Cover and refrigerate for at least 1 hour to marinate. In the meantime, soak 12–16 bamboo skewers in water to prevent them from burning during cooking.

2. In a food processor, combine the remaining 1/2 cup coconut milk, 1 tbsp. lime juice, Thai chili pepper and cashews and process until smooth. Add additional lime juice as needed to form a creamy consistency.

3. Preheat the broiler or grill. Drain the chicken strips and discard the marinade. Drain the bamboo skewers. Thread 1 strip of chicken onto each skewer. Broil chicken skewers for 3 minutes, then turn and broil until just cooked through, about 1–2 minutes longer. Brush on the cashew sauce to serve.

Beef Skewers with Mustard and Scallions

Tender beef is briefly marinated to add flavor, then wrapped around scallions for a spicy skewered treat.

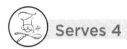 Serves 4

- 3 tbsps. extra virgin olive oil
- 2 tsps. minced garlic
- 1 tsp. ground mustard
- 1 tsp. smoked paprika
- 1 tbsp. crushed red pepperflakes

- 1 tsp. freshly ground black pepper
- 2 tbsps. lime juice
- 2 (8-oz.) beef tenderloins, halved and cut into 1-inch slices
- 12 scallions, trimmed and cut into 6-inch pieces

1. In a shallow bowl, whisk together the oil, garlic, mustard, paprika, pepper flakes, black pepper and lime juice. Add the beef strips and toss to coat. Cover, refrigerate and marinate for 30 minutes. In the meantime, soak 12–16 bamboo skewers in water to prevent them from burning during cooking.

2. Drain the beef strips and discard the marinade. Drain the bamboo skewers.

3. Set a slice of beef on a work surface and season with pepper. Arrange a scallion lengthwise on the meat and trim it flush with the meat. Roll up the meat around the scallion. Cut the rolls into approximately 1 1/2-inch pieces. Repeat with the remaining slices of beef scallions. Thread two pieces of rolled beef onto each skewer.

4. Preheat the broiler or grill. Broil the beef scallion skewers for 2 minutes, then turn and broil until just medium rare, about 1–2 minutes longer (2–3 minutes longer for medium to well done).

Chef's Tip: Save the green parts of the scallions to add flavor to broth-based soups.

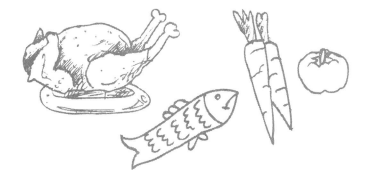

Green Vegetable Dip

Serve this simply delicious dip with celery and carrot sticks for a tasty snack.

 Serves 4

- ½ cup Mayonnaise (see recipe p. 54)
- ½ cup coconut milk
- 2 tbsps. lime juice
- 1 garlic clove, finely chopped
- 2 anchovy fillets, finely chopped
- ½ cup chopped fresh parsley
- ¼ cup roughly chopped fresh basil
- 4 scallions, trimmed and coarsely chopped
- ¼ tsp. cayenne pepper
- Freshly ground black pepper to taste

- Combine the mayonnaise, coconut milk and lime juice in a bowl. Stir in the remaining ingredients. Season with pepper to taste. Cover and refrigerate at least 1 hour to allow the flavors to combine.

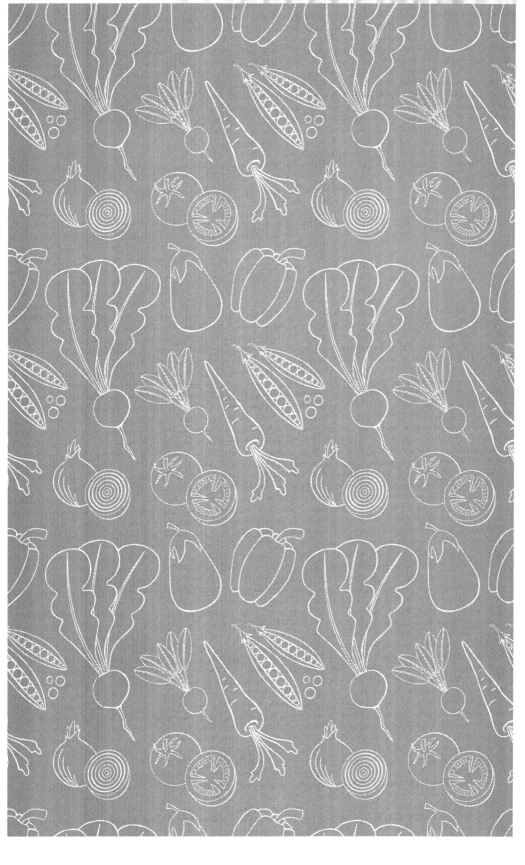

Chapter 6

Salads and Soups

- Roasted Beet Salad with Pomegranate and Pine Nuts
- Daikon, Carrot and Radish Salad
- Celery Root, Apples and Endive Salad with Poppy Seeds
- Baby Beet Greens and Watercress Salad with Pecans
- Quail with Belgian Endive and Blueberries
- Crab and Avocado Salad
- Spinach and Cantaloupe with Pine Nuts
- Asparagus and Belgian Endive with Walnuts
- Chicken and Pineapple Salad with Macadamia Nuts
- Shrimp, Zucchini and Tomato Soup
- Pumpkin Soup
- Carrot Ginger Soup
- Chicken Escarole Soup
- Asparagus Soup
- Red Pepper and Tomato Soup
- Butternut Squash and Apple Soup

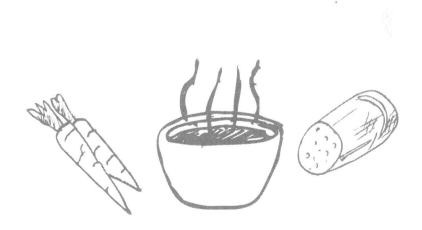

Roasted Beet Salad with Pomegranate and Pine Nuts

Warm roasted beets make a delicious salad with the addition of a savory dressing, tangy pomegranate seeds and toasted pine nuts.

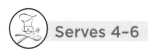 Serves 4-6

- 2 lbs. beets, tops and roots trimmed
- 1 tsp. finely chopped shallot
- 4 tbsps. extra virgin olive oil
- 1 tsp. freshly ground black pepper

- 2 tsps. lemon juice
- 2 tsps. chopped fresh mint
- Seeds from ½ pomegranate (approximately ¼ cup)
- ¼ cup toasted pine nuts

1. Preheat the oven to 375 degrees F. Line a baking sheet with aluminum foil and set aside.

2. Cut the beets into halves and place into a medium bowl. Toss the beets with the shallot, 2 tbsps. olive oil and freshly ground black pepper. Spoon beets onto the baking sheet and cover with foil. Place in the oven and roast for 45–60 minutes, until they are fork tender. Remove from the oven and uncover. Allow to cool slightly.

3. Combine the remaining 2 tbsps. olive oil and lemon juice. Return the beets to the bowl and toss with the olive oil and lemon juice mixture. Toss the beets with the fresh mint, pomegranate seeds and pine nuts and serve.

Chef's Tip: If you prefer the beets cold, roast them ahead of time when you are roasting other meats, etc. They will keep in the refrigerator for up to 3 days.

Daikon, Carrot and Radish Salad

Fresh root vegetables combine for a crunchy salad that's easily prepared ahead. Toasted sesame oil should only be consumed in small amounts on Paleo, but it packs a lot of flavor.

 Serve 4

- 3 tbsps. extra virgin olive oil
- 1 ½ tsps. toasted sesame oil
- 1 tbsp. lemon juice
- 1 tsp. fresh ginger, minced
- 1 tsp. finely chopped shallot
- 1 tsp. lemon zest
- 1 daikon, peeled and shaved into ribbons

- 8 small radishes, peeled and sliced thin
- 8 baby carrots, cut lengthwise into thin strips
- 2 cups diced cucumber
- 2 tsps. fresh chopped dill
- 1 tsp. sesame seeds

- Whisk together the olive oil, sesame oil, lemon juice, ginger, shallot and lemon zest and set aside. In a medium bowl, toss together the daikon, radishes, carrots and cucumber. Toss with dressing. Sprinkle with dill and sesame seeds to serve.

Chef's Tip: Radishes can differ in how peppery they taste (French breakfast radishes tend to be the mildest), but all radish varieties can turn pungent when grown in hot weather.

Celery Root, Apples and Endive Salad with Poppy Seeds

The gnarly appearance of celery root belies its elegant taste. The cut celery root may be refrigerated in the lemon juice water mixture until ready to serve.

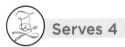 **Serves 4**

- 1 medium celery root, peeled and cut into matchstick-size strips
- 4 tbsps. lemon juice
- 1 tsp. ground mustard
- ½ tsp. minced garlic
- ⅓ cup avocado oil
- 2 tsps. poppy seeds
- 2 tart apples (like Granny Smith) peeled and cut into matchstick-size strips
- 2 heads Belgian endive, ends trimmed and cut lengthwise into thin strips

1. Fill a large bowl with ice water and stir in 2 tbsps. lemon juice. Add the cut celery root and allow to soak for 12–15 minutes. Drain completely and pat celery root dry.

2. In a large bowl, whisk together the ground mustard, 2 tbsps. lemon juice and garlic. Gradually drizzle in the avocado oil, whisking constantly to incorporate it. Whisk in the poppy seeds.

3. Add the celery root, apple and endive strips to the bowl and toss with the dressing to serve.

Baby Beet Greens and Watercress Salad with Pecans

Quality ingredients shine in this simple yet sophisticated salad.

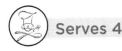 Serves 4

- 3 tbsps. extra virgin olive oil
- 1 tbsp. lemon juice
- 1 tsp. minced shallot

- 3 cups baby beet greens
- 2 bunches watercress, stems removed
- ¼ cup toasted pecans

- In a medium bowl, whisk together the olive oil, lemon juice and shallot. Add the beet greens and watercress and toss to combine. Sprinkle on pecans to serve.

Quail with Belgian Endive and Blueberries

This elegant dish takes minutes to prepare.

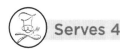 Serves 4

- ¼ cup plus 3 tbsps. extra virgin olive oil
- 1 tsp. minced garlic
- 4 semi-boneless quail
- Freshly ground black pepper

- 2 heads Belgian endive, leaves separated
- 2 tbsps. lemon juice
- ½ cup blueberries
- Preheat a grill or broiler.

- Combine 2 tbsps. olive oil with the garlic and brush all over the quail. Season the quail with pepper. Grill the quail until lightly browned and cooked through, about 4–5 minutes per side. Keep warm and allow to rest 5 minutes. In the meantime, heat 1 tbsp. olive oil in a large skillet over medium heat. Add the endive and cook until just wilted, about 1–1 1/2 minutes. Remove the endive to a warm plate. Heat the remaining 1/4 cup olive oil in the skillet. Stir in the lemon juice and blueberries and cook for 1 minute. Divide the endive among 4 plates and place a grilled quail on each. Spoon the warm blueberry dressing over the quail to serve.

Chef's Tip: Semi-boneless quail have the all bones except the wings and lower legs removed. They are also delicious stuffed with apples, cranberries and sausage and roasted in the oven for 20–25 minutes. D'Artagnan is an excellent source for quail and other game.

Crab and Avocado Salad

Delicious fresh crab and creamy avocado come together in a simply elegant dish.

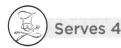 Serves 4

- 3 tbsps. Mayonnaise (see recipe p. 54)
- ½ tsp. ground mustard
- 1 tbsp. lemon juice
- 2 tsps. chopped fresh dill
- Freshly ground pepper to taste
- ½ lb. fresh lump crabmeat

- 1 avocado, peeled, seeded and diced
- 1 tsp. lime juice
- 2 cups arugula (or other salad greens)
- 3 tbsps. avocado oil
- 2 tbsps. fresh chopped chives

- In a small bowl, whisk together the mayonnaise, mustard and 1 tbsp. lemon juice. Stir in the fresh dill. Season with pepper. Gently stir in the crabmeat until combined. In a separate bowl, toss the avocado with the lime juice. Divide the arugula evenly among four plates. Mix the avocado oil with the remaining 1 tbsp. lemon juice and drizzle the avocado oil over the arugula. Divide the avocado evenly among the plates and mound in the center. Mound the crab meat evenly on top of the avocado. Sprinkle with fresh chives to serve.

Spinach and Cantaloupe with Pine Nuts

Sweet ripe cantaloupe is the perfect match for fresh spinach. The pine nuts add texture to this refreshing summer salad.

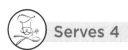 Serves 4

- ⅓ cup extra virgin olive oil
- 1 shallot, peeled and finely chopped
- ½ cup chopped flat-leaf parsley
- 2 tbsps. lemon juice
- 10 oz. baby spinach, stems removed
- ½ small cantaloupe, peeled, seeded and cut into ½-inch cubes
- ½ cup toasted pine nuts

- Whisk together the olive oil, shallot, parsley and lemon juice in a medium bowl. Add the spinach and toss to coat. Add the cantaloupe and pine nuts to serve.

Asparagus and Belgian Endive with Walnuts

The blend of textures adds a layer of interest to a tasty salad combination.

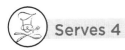 Serves 4

- 3 tbsps. extra virgin olive oil
- 1 tsp. minced shallot
- 1 tbsp. lemon juice
- 1 tsp. chopped chives
- Freshly ground pepper to taste
- 2 heads Belgian endive, trimmed and leaves separated
- 20 medium asparagus spears, trimmed and blanched until just cooked through
- 1 tbsp. walnut or avocado oil
- ¼ cup coarsely chopped toasted walnuts

- In a large bowl, whisk together the olive oil, shallot, lemon juice and chives. Season with pepper to taste. Add the endive leaves and toss to coat. Divide the endive evenly among four plates. Place 5 asparagus spears on top of each plate. Drizzle the asparagus with the walnut oil. Sprinkle on the walnuts to serve.

Chef's Tip: Asparagus may be prepared up to a day ahead and refrigerated until ready to serve.

Chicken and Pineapple Salad with Macadamia Nuts

The chicken may be poached or grilled for this tropical salad.

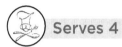 Serves 4

- ¼ cup mayonnaise
- 2 tbsps. lemon juice
- ¼ cup chopped flat-leaf parsley
- ¼ tsp. cayenne pepper
- Freshly ground pepper to taste
- 2 (6- to 8-oz.) boneless skinless chicken breasts, fully cooked and cut into bite-size pieces

- 1 pineapple, peeled, cored and cut into 1-inch chunks
- 3 tbsps. unsweetened coconut flakes
- 2 cups fresh mixed greens
- ½ cup chopped macadamia nuts

- In a large bowl, combine the mayonnaise, lemon juice, parsley and cayenne pepper. Season with pepper to taste. Add the chicken and toss to coat evenly. Toss the pineapple chunks with the coconut and add to the salad. Divide the greens among 4 plates. Divide the chicken salad evenly and sprinkle with the macadamia nuts to serve.

Chef's Tip: Prepare the chicken breasts ahead while cooking another meal and refrigerate until ready to serve.

Shrimp, Zucchini and Tomato Soup

Tomato and zucchini bring a summery flavor to this easily prepared soup.

 Serves 4

- 3 tbsps. extra virgin olive oil
- 1 pound medium shrimp, about 24–30 (shelled and deveined)
- 1 cup sliced onion
- 1 tsp. minced garlic
- 2 medium zucchini, peeled and cut into ½-inch dice

- 2 cups diced tomatoes
- 3 cups Fish Stock (see Recipe p. 46) or Chicken Stock (see Recipe p. 42)
- 2 tsps. crushed red pepper flakes
- 2 tbsps. lime juice
- ½ cup shredded basil
- Freshly ground pepper to taste

- Heat a large saucepan or Dutch oven over medium-high heat. Add 1 tbsp. olive oil and stir in the shrimp. Cook until just pink, about 2–3 minutes. Turn to cook other side, about 1–2 minutes longer. Remove the shrimp to a bowl and keep warm. Heat the remaining 2 tbsps. olive oil. Add the onion and cook until it begins to soften, about 4–5 minutes. Add the garlic and cook 30 seconds longer. Add the zucchini and tomatoes, and cook for 2–3 minutes. Pour in the stock and bring to a boil. Lower to a simmer and add the pepper flakes. Simmer for 5 minutes. Remove from the heat and add the shrimp. Stir in the lime juice and basil. Season with freshly ground pepper to serve.

Chef's Tip: If preparing the soup ahead of time, do not add the shrimp, as they will toughen when reheated. Reheat the tomato zucchini base and then cook and add the shrimp just before serving.

Pumpkin Soup

Crunchy pumpkin seeds add a little texture to this creamy soup.

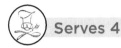 **Serves 4**

- 3 tbsps. extra virgin olive oil
- 1 lb. fresh pumpkin, peeled, seeded and cubed
- 1 small onion, finely chopped
- 2 cups Chicken Stock (see Recipe p. 42)
- 1 cup coconut milk
- ¼ tsp. cayenne pepper
- 2 tbsps. chopped flat-leaf parsley
- Freshly ground pepper to taste
- 3 tbsps. toasted shelled pumpkin seeds

- Heat the olive oil in a large skillet over medium-high heat. Add the pumpkin and onions and lower the heat. Sauté until the pumpkin is softened, about 5 minutes. Pour in 1 cup of chicken stock and continue cooking until the pumpkin is very soft, about 10 minutes. Let cool slightly. Working in batches, puree in a blender until smooth. Spoon the mixture into a medium saucepan or Dutch oven and stir in the remaining 1 cup of chicken stock, plus the coconut milk and cayenne pepper. Bring to a simmer and cook for 5 minutes. Stir in the parsley and season with pepper to taste. Sprinkle with pumpkin seeds to serve.

Carrot Ginger Soup

Sweet potato adds to the creamy texture of this ginger-scented soup.

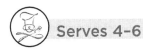 **Serves 4-6**

- 2 tbsps. extra virgin olive oil
- ½ cup minced onion
- 2 tbsps. minced fresh ginger
- 3 ½ cups Chicken Stock (see Recipe p. 42)
- 4 cups peeled baby carrots (about 1 ½ pounds), cut into 1-inch pieces
- 1 large sweet potato, peeled and diced
- 1 cup coconut milk
- ¼ tsp. ground curry powder
- ½ tsp. cayenne pepper
- ¼ cup sliced toasted almonds

1. Heat oil in heavy large saucepan or cast iron Dutch oven over medium-high heat. Add onion and ginger and sauté until onion is translucent, about 5 minutes. Add chicken stock, carrots and sweet potato. Cover and simmer until carrots and potatoes are tender, about 30 minutes.

2. Working in batches, puree mixture in blender or processor. Return soup to saucepan. Stir in coconut milk. Stir in curry powder and cayenne pepper. Cook over low heat for 5 minutes. Season the soup to taste with freshly ground pepper. Top soup with almonds to serve.

Chicken Escarole Soup

Escarole is a healthy and flavorful addition to this stock-based soup.

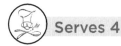 **Serves 4**

- 1 tbsp. extra virgin olive oil
- 1 leek, white parts only, thinly sliced into rings
- 3 carrots, peeled and cut into ½-inch chunks
- 4 cups Chicken Stock (see Recipe p. 42)
- 4 scallions, ends removed and sliced into 1/2-inch rounds
- 1 cup shredded cooked chicken breast
- 3 cups escarole, thoroughly washed and stems removed
- 2 eggs
- 1 tsp. lime juice
- ¼ cup chopped fresh Italian parsley
- 10 chives, finely chopped
- Freshly ground black pepper to taste

- Heat the olive oil over medium heat in a heavy stock pot or cast iron Dutch oven. Stir in the leeks and cook until softened, stirring constantly, about 4–5 minutes. Add the carrots and stir just to coat. Pour in the broth. Bring just to a boil, then lower heat to a simmer and cover. Simmer until carrots are tender, about 20–25 minutes. Add the scallions and chicken and simmer for 5 more minutes. Add the escarole all at once and cook until just limp. Remove from heat. Whisk the eggs in a measuring cup until scrambled. Pour in the eggs and stir until combined. Stir in the lime juice and herbs. Season with freshly cracked pepper and serve warm.

Chef's Tip: Baby spinach may be substituted for escarole. For an added layer of flavor, cook the chicken breasts in the stock the night before making this soup. Remove the chicken and refrigerate it and the stock overnight, skimming any fat off the surface before using.

Asparagus Soup

Fresh seasonal asparagus is the star of this simply delicious soup.

 Serves 4

- 2 tbsps. extra virgin olive oil
- 1 large onion, thinly sliced
- 1 tsp. minced garlic

- 1 ½ pounds asparagus, blanched
- 3 cups Chicken Stock (see Recipe p. 42)
- Freshly ground black pepper

- Heat olive oil in a large saucepan or Dutch oven on medium heat. Sauté onions until soft and translucent. Add garlic and cook 30 seconds longer. Add asparagus and chicken stock. Bring to a boil. Reduce heat and simmer for 20 minutes until asparagus are soft. Pour soup into a blender no more than half full. Working in batches, puree the soup with a blender (or use an immersion blender) until smooth. Season with freshly ground pepper to taste.

Red Pepper and Tomato Soup

Roasting bell peppers mellows their taste and concentrates their flavor.

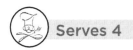 **Serves 4**

- 2 red bell peppers, seeds and stalks removed
- 2 tbsps. coconut oil
- ¼ cup chopped onion
- ¼ cup chopped celery
- 1 leek, white part only, coarsely chopped
- 1 tsp. minced garlic
- 10 plum tomatoes, peeled, seeded and coarsely chopped (or use 1 [28-ounce] can of tomatoes, preferably San Marzano)
- 2 cups Chicken Stock (see Recipe p. 42)
- 1 cup coconut milk
- Freshly ground black pepper

1. Roast the bell peppers over an open flame until the skins are charred (or roast on a baking sheet in a preheated 400 degree F. oven for 1 hour). Place the grilled peppers in a paper bag to steam and loosen the skin. Allow the peppers to cool in the bag for 5 minutes. Remove the peppers from the bag and rub off the skin with a paper towel. Coarsely chop the roasted peppers and set aside.

2. Heat coconut oil in a large saucepan or Dutch oven on medium heat. Sauté onions, celery, leeks and garlic until soft and translucent, about 4–5 minutes. Add tomatoes, roasted peppers and chicken stock and stir to combine. Bring to a boil. Reduce heat and simmer for 20 minutes. Stir in coconut milk and simmer for 5 minutes. Pour soup into a blender no more than half full. Working in batches, puree the soup with a blender (or use an immersion blender) until smooth. Season with black pepper to serve.

Butternut Squash and Apple Soup

Roasting the butternut squash accentuates the flavors of autumn in this hearty soup.

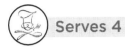 Serves 4

- 2 butternut squash, peeled, seeded and cut into 2-inch pieces
- 3 tart apples (e.g., Granny Smith), peeled, seeded and cut into quarters
- 2 tbsps. extra virgin olive oil
- 4 cups Chicken Stock (see Recipe p. 42)
- 2 tbsps. coconut oil
- ½ cup chopped onion
- 2 tbsps. minced fresh ginger
- 1 tsp. ground cinnamon
- 1 cup coconut cream (optional)
- ½ tsp. freshly grated nutmeg
- Freshly ground black pepper to taste

1. Preheat the oven to 350 degrees F. Line a roasting pan or baking sheet with foil.

2. Place the squash and apples into the roasting pan and drizzle with the oil. Roast for 30–40 minutes, until tender. Combine the squash and apples with 1 cup of chicken stock in a food processor or blender and process until smooth.

3. Heat the coconut oil in a medium saucepan over medium-high heat. Add the onion and ginger, lower heat and cook for 2 minutes. Whisk in the squash apple puree, the remaining 3 cups stock and the cinnamon. Bring to a simmer. If you prefer a creamier consistency, add the coconut cream and stir to combine. Season with nutmeg and pepper to serve.

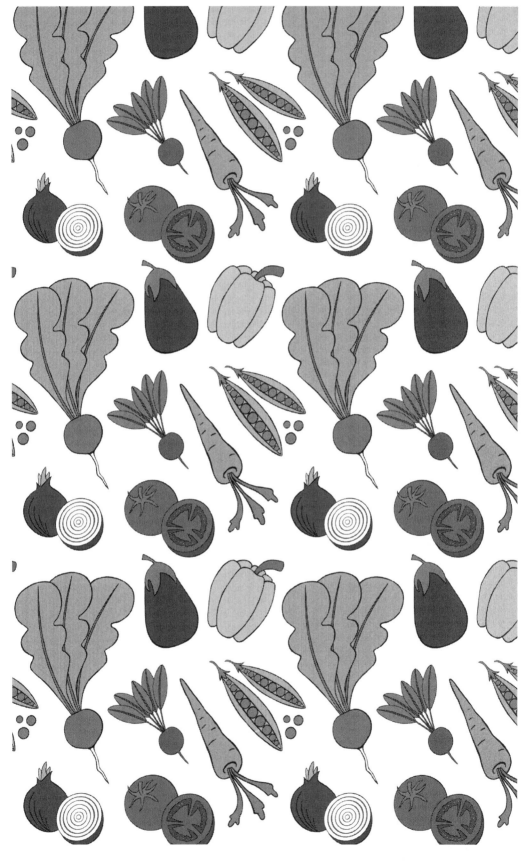

Chapter 7

Entrees

- Tuna with Anchovies, Tomatoes and Fennel
- Shrimp with Almonds and Mango Salsa
- Chicken with Tomatoes, Peppers and Spinach
- Shrimp and Pineapple Stir Fry
- Beef with Carrots and Mushrooms
- Chicken with Mushrooms and Tomatoes
- Seafood Stew
- Shrimp with Paprika and Scallions
- Braised Short Ribs
- Root Vegetables and Turkey Stew
- Buffalo Chili with Butternut Squash
- Pork Chops with Apples

- Caramelized Duck Breasts with Blueberries
- Codfish with Dill
- Halibut with Zucchini and Scallions
- Salmon with Sweet Onions, Mustard and Rosemary
- Braised Veal Shanks
- Trout with Lemon and Pine Nuts
- Sea Scallops with Green Curry and Zucchini
- Flank Steak with Cilantro and Mint
- Salmon with Shitakes and Scallions
- Rack of Lamb with Mint Pesto and Pecans
- Venison Medallions with Apple, Pear and Cranberries

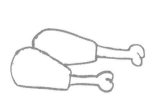
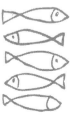
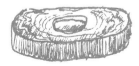

Tuna with Anchovies, Tomatoes and Fennel

This Provencal-inspired dish is quick to prepare and serve.

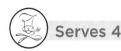 **Serves 4**

- 3 ½ tbsps. extra virgin olive oil
- 1 cup finely chopped onion
- 2 tsps. minced garlic
- 1 fennel bulb, trimmed and thinly sliced
- 8 plum tomatoes, coarsely cut into ½-inch cubes (seeds and skin removed)
- ¼ cup Fish Stock (see Recipe p. 46) or Chicken Stock (see Recipe p. 42)
- 2 tsps. fresh thyme leaves
- 4 (4- to 6-oz.) pieces of tuna filet, about 1 inch thick
- 2 tsps. freshly ground black pepper
- 8 anchovy filets, packed in oil (not salt)
- 2 tsps. chopped fresh Italian parsley
- 2 tsps. minced lemon zest

1. Preheat the oven to 350 degrees F.

2. Heat 3 tbsps. of the olive oil in a medium skillet over medium heat. Add the onion and garlic and cook until just softened, about 2 minutes. Stir in the fennel and cook for 2–3 minutes longer. Stir in the tomatoes and thyme. Add the stock and bring to a boil. Lower to a simmer and cook for 5–7 minutes, until tomatoes are softened. Remove from the heat.

3. Brush the remaining olive oil onto the bottom of a casserole or Dutch oven large enough to accommodate the tuna. Place the pieces of tuna into the casserole. Sprinkle on the black pepper. Cook for 1–2 minutes until just seared. Turn and cook the other side 1 minute longer. Pour the tomato mixture over the tuna. Arrange the anchovies evenly over the top. Bake for 8–10 minutes, until tuna is tender and medium rare (5–8 minutes longer for medium to well done).

4. Remove from oven and cool slightly. Sprinkle with parsley and lemon zest to serve.

Chef's Tip: Substitute 1 (28-oz.) can of tomatoes with their liquid for the fresh tomatoes and stock if desired.

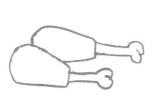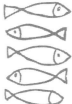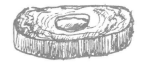

Shrimp with Almonds and Mango Salsa

Look for unsalted Marcona almonds roasted with olive oil for this crunchy shrimp dish.

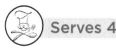 **Serves 4**

- 1 mango, peeled and diced
- 1 jalapeno, seeded and finely chopped
- 3 tbsps. chopped red onion
- 2 tbsps. lime juice
- 1 tbsp. chopped cilantro
- Freshly ground black pepper to taste

- ¼ cup almond flour
- 1 tsp. cayenne pepper
- 1 tsp. smoked paprika
- 1 cup Marcona almonds, coarsely chopped
- 1 large egg, beaten
- 20 jumbo shrimp, peeled and deveined

1. Combine the mango, jalapeno, red onion, lime juice and cilantro and mix well. Season with pepper to taste. Refrigerate covered until ready to serve.

2. Heat the oven to 400 degrees F. Line a baking sheet with parchment. Set an oven-proof baking rack on top.

3. Place the flour into a shallow bowl and mix in the cayenne pepper and paprika. Place the chopped almonds onto a plate or into a shallow bowl. Whisk the egg lightly in a small bowl. Dredge each shrimp through the flour mixture, then the egg, and finally through the almonds until well coated. Arrange shrimp on the baking rack. Bake for 8–10 minutes, until lightly browned and cooked through. Serve shrimp with mango salsa.

Chef's Tip: If you don't have a baking rack, turn the shrimp after 6 minutes to brown the other side.

Chicken with Tomatoes, Peppers and Spinach

Bone-in chicken breasts require a longer cooking time but will yield a moist dish with complex flavors.

 Serves 4

- ¼ cup extra virgin olive oil
- 4 bone-in skinless chicken breast halves
- 1 red or yellow bell pepper, sliced into ¼-inch strips
- 1 cup sliced onion
- 2 cloves garlic, chopped
- 2 cups diced plum tomatoes
- 1 tsp. crushed red pepper flakes
- ½ cup red wine (optional)

- ½ cup Chicken Stock (see Recipe p. 42)
- 1 tbsp. fresh chopped thyme
- 1 tbsp. fresh chopped oregano
- 4 cups baby spinach, stems removed
- ¼ cup chopped fresh flat-leaf parsley
- Freshly ground black pepper to taste

- In a large skillet or Dutch oven, heat the olive oil over medium heat. When the oil is hot, cook the chicken until browned on both sides. Remove from the pan and set aside. Add the peppers and onion and cook until softened, about 4–5 minutes. Add the garlic and cook for 1 minute. Add the tomatoes, red pepper flakes and wine (if using). Scrape any bits off the bottom of the pan. Return the chicken to the pan, add the stock and bring the mixture to a boil. Stir in the thyme and oregano. Reduce the heat and simmer, covered, until the chicken is cooked through, about 20–30 minutes. Add the baby spinach and stir until it is just wilted. Remove from heat. Sprinkle with the parsley and season with black pepper to serve.

Chef's Tip: If you substitute boneless chicken breasts, reduce the cooking time to 10–15 minutes.

Shrimp and Pineapple Stir Fry

This combination of flavor and texture yields a satisfying stir fry without the rice.

 Serves 4

- 2 large eggs
- 3 tbsps. coconut oil
- 1 lb. extra-large shrimp, peeled and deveined (about 20 shrimp)
- 1 cup sliced sweet onion
- 1 cup sliced mushrooms
- 3 scallions, trimmed and thinly sliced
- 1 tsp. minced garlic

- 1 Thai chili pepper, seeded and minced
- 1 cup diced fresh pineapple
- 1 cup bean sprouts
- 2 tsps. crushed red pepper flakes
- 2 tbsps. lime juice
- ¼ cup toasted almonds, coarsely chopped
- ¼ cup chopped cilantro

1. In a small bowl or measuring cup, whisk the eggs together. Heat 1 tbsp. coconut in a medium skillet over medium heat. Pour in the eggs and swirl to coat the bottom of the pan (as if making an omelet). Cook until just set, then flip egg to cook the other side. Remove the egg from the pan and place on a cutting board. Cut the egg into thin strips and set aside.

2. Heat 1 tbsp. coconut oil in a large skillet or wok over medium-high heat. Add the shrimp and cook until starting to brown, about 1–2 minutes. Flip the shrimp and cook until pink and opaque, about 1–2 minutes longer. Remove from the pan and set aside.

3. Add the remaining 1 tbsp. of coconut oil to the pan. Add the onions and mushrooms and cook until soft, about 3–4 minutes. Stir in the scallions and cook 1 minute longer. Stir in the minced garlic and Thai pepper and cook for 30 seconds. Stir in the shrimp and cook 1 minute longer.

4. Remove from heat and stir in the pineapple, bean sprouts, pepper flakes and lime juice. Stir in the reserved egg strips. Garnish with toasted almonds and cilantro to serve.

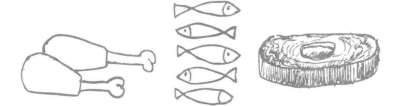

Beef with Carrots and Mushrooms

A Paleo version of the classic French dish Beef Bourguignon is easy to prepare ahead of time and tastes delicious the next day too.

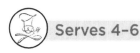 **Serves 4-6**

- 3 lbs. chuck steak or beef blade
- Freshly ground black pepper
- 4 tbsps. extra virgin olive oil
- 1 cup sliced onions
- 1 leek, coarsely chopped
- 2 shallots, peeled and coarsely chopped
- 4 large carrots, peeled and sliced diagonally into 1-inch chunks
- 4 garlic cloves, 2 crushed and 2 chopped
- 1 cup red wine (optional)

- 3 cups Beef Stock (see Recipe p. 44)
- 1 cup plum tomatoes, seeded, peeled and chopped
- Bouquet garni (sprig of parsley, thyme, rosemary and 2 bay leaves tied together with butcher's twine or in cheesecloth)
- 1 tsp. fresh thyme leaves
- 1 lb. fresh mushrooms, stems discarded, caps thickly sliced
- ½ cup chopped fresh parsley, optional

1. Preheat the oven to 325 degrees F.

2. Cut the meat into 1 1/2-inch cubes and trim away any excess fat. Pat dry. Season with freshly ground black pepper. Heat 2 tbsps. olive oil in a large Dutch oven. Add the meat and sauté until all sides are lightly browned, about 4–5 minutes. Pour meat and any rendered liquid into a bowl and set aside. Return Dutch oven to medium heat and add 2 tbsps. Olive oil. Add the onions and cook for 4–5 minutes until beginning to soften. Add the leek, shallots, 1 carrot and 2 crushed garlic cloves. Add the wine (if using) and allow to reduce into half. Add the beef stock. Add the bouquet garni and bring to a boil. Add the reserved meat and liquid and return to a boil. Cover and lower to a simmer.

3. Place in the oven for about 2 hours or until the meat and vegetables are very tender when pierced with a fork. Remove from the oven and remove and discard the bouquet garni. Strain the liquid into a medium saucepan, reserving the meat and vegetables. Return the liquid to low heat and reduce the liquid until thickened to the desired consistency. Return the vegetables, meat and reduced sauce to the Dutch oven. Bring to a simmer and keep warm.

4. Heat the remaining 1 tbsp. olive oil in a medium skillet over medium-high heat. Add the mushrooms and sauté for 8–10 minutes until lightly browned and cooked through. Stir the mushrooms into the stew. Season with parsley to serve.

Chef's Tip: This dishes freezes well, so consider making double the amount. Freeze the mixture in individual portions for a simple, savory take-along lunch.

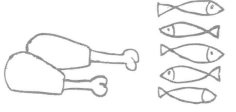
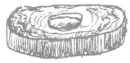

Chicken with Mushrooms and Tomatoes

Tarragon adds a complex flavor with hints of fennel, licorice and mint.

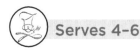 **Serves 4-6**

- 6 small bone-in chicken breasts
- 6 chicken wings
- 4 tbsps. extra virgin olive oil
- 2 shallots, finely chopped
- 2 cup mushrooms, cleaned and sliced
- ¾ cup white wine (optional)

- 3 plum tomatoes, peeled, seeded and quartered
- 1 cup Chicken Stock (see Recipe p. 42)
- 2 tsps. chopped fresh tarragon
- 1 tsp. chopped fresh thyme
- 1 tsp. chopped fresh parsley

1. Heat 2 tbsps. olive oil in a large Dutch oven over medium-high heat. Add the chicken and sauté in batches on both sides until browned. Put on a baking sheet and cover with foil to keep. Pour the excess fat out of the pan and reserve for other uses if desired.

2. Heat the remaining olive oil in the Dutch oven. Add the shallots and cook until softened but not browned, about 3–4 minutes. Add the mushrooms and cook, stirring often, for about 3 minutes. Stir in the white wine (if using) and bring just to a boil. Stir in the tomatoes and stock. Bring to a boil, reduce the heat and add the tarragon and thyme. Return the chicken to the pan, cover and simmer for 30 minutes or until the chicken is tender and cooked through. Sprinkle with parsley to serve.

Chef's Tip: Reserve the rendered chicken fat to add flavor to chicken liver pate.

Seafood Stew

The Paleo version of another French classic, Bouillabaisse, is delicious and satisfying. Having your ingredients measured before cooking (referred to as "mis en place" or "putting in place" in professional kitchens) will ease the preparation. Marinating the fish for at least 2 hours adds a level of complexity to the dish.

 Serves 4

- ¼ tsp. saffron
- 2 tsps. lemon juice
- ¼ tsp. cayenne pepper
- 3 garlic cloves, peeled and minced
- 1 tsp. ground mustard
- 1 large egg yolk
- ¾ cup plus 8 tbsps. extra virgin olive oil
- 2 lbs. non-oily white fish, like sea bass, grouper or halibut, cut into 2-inch chunks
- 8 cloves garlic, chopped and divided in half
- 1 large fennel bulb
- 1 cup leeks, julienned

- ½ cup white wine (optional)
- 3 cups Fish Stock (see Recipe p. 46)
- 3 cups tomatoes, peeled, seeded and coarsely chopped
- ½ tsp. lemon zest
- 2 sprigs thyme, 1 bay leaf and 1 sprig rosemary, tied in a bundle
- ½ lb. dry sea scallops
- ½ lb. littleneck clams, scrubbed
- ½ lb. mussels, scrubbed and debearded
- 1 lb. large shrimp (20–25), peeled and deveined
- 2 tbsps. fresh parsley, coarsely chopped
- Freshly ground pepper to taste

1. Stir a pinch of the saffron into 1 tsp. lemon juice. In a food processor (or whisk), combine the cayenne pepper, garlic and mustard with the egg yolk and 1 tbsp. water and process until smooth. With the machine running (or whisking constantly), gradually drizzle in 3/4 cup olive oil to form a smooth emulsion. Add the lemon juice saffron

mixture and pulse to combine. Season with pepper and refrigerate until ready to use.

2. Marinate the fish. Lay the pieces of fish on a baking dish or sheet pan and sprinkle on 1/2 of the garlic. Remove the fennel fronds from the fennel and reserve the bulb. Layer on the fennel fronds. Drizzle with 4 tbsps. olive oil. Cover with plastic and place into the refrigerator. Marinate for at least 2 hours, turning the fish several times.

3. Remove the fish from the marinade when ready to prepare the stew. Slice the fennel bulb into thin strips. Heat the remaining 4 tbsps. of olive oil in a stock pot or Dutch oven over medium heat. Add the remaining 4 cloves of garlic and cook for 1 minute. Add the leeks and fennel and cook for 4–5 minutes, until softened. Add the white wine all at once (if using) and reduce by 1/3. Add the fish stock and bring to a boil. Add the tomatoes, lemon zest, herb bundle and the remaining saffron and lemon juice. Bring to a boil, then simmer for 5 minutes. Add the fish and scallops and cook for about 4–5 minutes longer, until almost cooked through. Add the clams and mussels and cover. Cook until the clams and mussels have just opened. Discard any unopened clams and mussels. Add the shrimp and cook 1–2 minutes longer until pink and just cooked through. Remove from heat. Remove the thyme bundle and discard. Sprinkle on the parsley and adjust the seasoning to taste.

4. Spoon the stew evenly into bowls. Serve with the mustard aioli to stir into the stew.

Chef's Tip: Chicken stock may be substituted for the fish stock if fish stock is unavailable.

Shrimp with Paprika and Scallions

A spicy New Orleans-style shrimp dish that's delicious served over sautéed spinach.

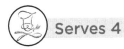 Serves 4

- ½ cup extra virgin olive oil
- 1 cup chopped scallions
- 2 tsps. minced garlic
- 1 ½ lbs. extra-large shrimp (15–20 per lb.), peeled and deveined
- 4 tsps. chopped fresh basil
- 4 tsps. chopped fresh thyme
- 4 tsps. chopped fresh parsley
- 1 bay leaf
- 4 tbsps. smoked paprika
- 2 tsps. cayenne pepper
- 2 tsps. freshly ground black pepper
- 1 tbsp. almond flour
- 1 cup white wine (optional)
- ¼ cup Fish Stock (see Recipe p. 46)
- 3 tsps. lemon juice

- Heat the olive oil in a Dutch oven or large skillet over medium-high heat. Add the chopped scallions and garlic and sauté for 1 minute. Add the shrimp all at once, stirring constantly to coat with oil. Add the fresh herbs, bay leaf, paprika, cayenne and black pepper and stir to combine, about 2 minutes. Stir in the almond flour and cook for 1 minute. Add the white wine (if using) and bring to a boil for 2–3 minutes. Add the fish stock and stir until liquid is reduced and mixture is thickened. Stir in the lemon juice and remove from heat to serve.

Braised Short Ribs

This dish is even better when made the day before and refrigerated overnight. Skim off any fat and reheat when ready to serve.

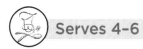 **Serves 4-6**

- 1 bottle dry red wine (optional)
- 6 bone-in short ribs – 7-8 oz. each (or 12 smaller ones)
- Freshly ground black pepper for seasoning
- 2 tbsps. almond flour
- 8 cloves garlic, peeled
- 2 medium carrots, peeled and cut into 1-inch lengths
- 2 stalks celery, trimmed and cut into 1-inch lengths

- 8 shallots, peeled and trimmed
- 1 medium leek, white parts only, thoroughly washed and cut into 1-inch lengths
- 6 sprigs Italian parsley
- 2 sprigs thyme
- 2 bay leaves
- 4 plum tomatoes, seeded and quartered
- 5–6 cups Beef Stock (see Recipe p. 44)

1. If using the wine, pour it into a large saucepan set over medium heat till it's hot but not boiling. Remove from the heat and carefully set it aflame. Return to heat and cook until the flames die out. Lower to a simmer and cook until reduced by half. Remove from heat.

2. Preheat the oven to 350 degrees F.

3. Season the ribs all over with pepper and sprinkle with the almond flour. Heat the oil over medium heat in a Dutch oven. Add the ribs and sear for 4–5 minutes per side, until browned all over. Transfer the browned ribs to a plate and continue in batches until all are done. Add the garlic, carrots, celery, shallots and leek and cook until lightly browned, about 6–7 minutes. Add the herbs, bay leaf and tomatoes and stir for 1 minute longer. Add the reduced wine (if using). Add the browned ribs to the pot. Add the beef stock until the ribs are just

covered. Bring to a boil, cover tightly with the lid and place the pan into the oven. After 1 hour, lift the lid and skim off any fat that has come to the surface. Braise for 1 1/2 hours longer (for a total of 2 1/2 hours), until the ribs are tender. (If you are making this recipe the night before, allow the ribs to cool in the pan and refrigerate overnight).

4. Transfer the meat to a warm platter and carefully remove any bones without shredding the meat. Bring the pan liquid to a boil and allow the liquid to reduce until slightly thickened (about 10–20 minutes). Pass through a fine mesh strainer and discard the solids. Season with pepper to taste. Serve the warm meat with roasted vegetables or over celery root puree.

Root Vegetable and Turkey Stew

In this hearty stew, boneless skinless turkey breast is added for a rich flavor. This Paleo version of cassoulet substitutes turkey for the traditional duck confit and omits the beans without sacrificing flavor.

 Serves 4-6

- 4 tbsps. extra virgin olive oil
- ½ onion, peeled, trimmed and diced
- 3 cloves garlic, peeled and finely chopped
- 3 plum tomatoes, 2 seeded and coarsely chopped, 1 seeded and quartered
- Freshly ground pepper to taste
- 6 stalks celery, trimmed and cut into 2-inch lengths
- 3 medium carrots, peeled, trimmed and cut into 2-inch lengths
- 2 large turnips, peeled, trimmed, halved lengthwise and cut into 2-inch lengths
- 1 medium fennel bulb, trimmed, halved and cut into 2-inch pieces
- 2 turkey breast halves, skinned, deboned and cut into cubes
- 3 cups Chicken Stock (see Recipe p. 42)
- Bouquet garni (3 sprigs Italian parsley, 2 sprigs sage and 2 sprigs thyme, tied together with kitchen twine)
- ¼ cup coconut flour
- 1 tbsp. coconut oil
- 1 large egg
- ¼ cup chopped parsley

1. Heat 2 tbsps. olive oil in a Dutch oven over medium heat. Add the onion and cook until tender, about 5–6 minutes. Add the garlic and cook 30 seconds longer. Add the 2 chopped tomatoes and cook for 1 minute. Spoon the mixture into a bowl, season with freshly ground pepper and set aside. Add the remaining 2 tbsps. olive oil to the pan over medium-high heat. Add the celery, carrots, turnips, fennel, and quartered tomato. Stir until beginning to soften, about 4–5 minutes. Add the turkey meat and sauté for 2–3 minutes. Add the chicken stock

to the pan and bring to a boil. Add the bouquet garni. Lower the heat to a simmer and cook until the vegetables are tender and liquid is reduced in half, about 30 minutes.

2. When the vegetables are almost done, preheat the oven to 375 degrees F.

3. Remove the pan from the heat. Discard the bouquet garni and whatever is left of the tomato. Spoon on the tomato onion mixture. Place the lid on and cook in the oven for 15 minutes. In a small bowl, toss the coconut flour with the coconut oil with a pastry blender or fork. Mix in the egg and parsley until combined and mixture is crumbly. Remove the lid from the Dutch oven and sprinkle with the crumb mixture. Return to the oven uncovered and cook for 10–12 minutes more, until the crumbs are golden brown and crusty. Serve immediately.

Chef's Tip: Leftover roast turkey is a delicious substitute (if it's available).

Buffalo Chili with Butternut Squash

Butternut squash adds texture to this satisfying chili dish.

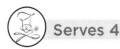 **Serves 4**

- 1 avocado, peeled, seeded and coarsely chopped
- 2 tbsps. lime juice
- 3 tbsps. extra virgin olive oil
- 1 lb. ground buffalo
- 1 medium onion, chopped
- 1 tsp. minced garlic
- 10 plum tomatoes, peeled, seeded and chopped
- 2 jalapeno peppers, seeded and chopped
- 1 serrano pepper, seeded and chopped
- 1 tsp. ground cumin
- ¼ tsp. cayenne pepper
- 2 tbsps. Chili Powder (see p. 56)
- 1 tsp. crushed red pepper flakes
- 2 tsps. chopped fresh oregano
- 2 cups Beef Stock (see Recipe p. 44) or Chicken Stock (see Recipe p. 42)
- 1 ½–2 lbs. butternut squash, peeled, seeded and cut into ½-inch cubes (about 2 cups)
- Freshly ground black pepper to taste

1. In a small bowl, use the back of a fork to mash together the avocado and 1 tbsp. lime juice into a paste. Cover and refrigerate until ready to use.

2. Heat the olive oil in a Dutch oven over medium heat. Add the buffalo and cook until lightly browned, stirring to break up lumps. Add the onion and garlic and cook 2–3 minutes longer, until beginning to soften. Add the tomatoes, peppers, cumin, cayenne pepper, chili powder, pepper flakes and oregano and stir to combine. Stir in the stock and bring to a boil. Lower to a simmer and cook uncovered for about 45 minutes. Add the butternut squash and cook for 10–12 minutes longer, until squash is just tender (add water or more stock if needed). Stir in the remaining 1 tbsp. lime juice. Season with pepper to taste. Serve with the mashed avocado.

Chef's Tip: Substitute 1 lb. venison or mix both venison and buffalo for a delicious variation.

Pork Chops with Apples

Pork chops are stuffed with a savory apple filling and then roasted to combine the flavors.

 Serves 4

- 4 tbsps. extra virgin olive oil
- ½ cup chopped onion
- 1 tsp. minced garlic
- 6 oz. ground pork
- 2 green apples, peeled, cored and diced
- ½ tsp. chopped sage

- ½ tsp. chopped thyme
- ¼ cup coarsely ground almonds
- 4 (1 ½-inch thick) center-cut boneless pork chops (6–7 oz. each)
- Freshly ground black pepper to taste
- ½ cup Chicken Stock (see Recipe p. 42)

1. Preheat the oven to 375 degrees F.

2. Heat 2 tbsps. of the olive oil in a large skillet or Dutch oven over medium-high heat. Sauté the onion for 2–3 minutes, until just slightly softened. Add the garlic and sauté 30 seconds longer. Stir in the ground pork and cook for 3–4 minutes longer, stirring constantly to break up lumps. Add the apples, herbs and almonds and stir until heated through.

3. Remove the skillet from the heat and spoon the stuffing into a bowl. Return the skillet to medium-high heat and add the remaining 2 tbsps. olive oil. Season the chops with black pepper to taste. Add the chops and cook for 3–4 minutes until lightly browned. Turn the chops over and cook for 3–4 minutes longer. Remove the pan from the heat. Cool slightly. Divide the filling, using a tablespoon to carefully mound it into each chop. Arrange the chops with cut side facing the center so if any filling comes out, it can be easily scooped with each chop. Return the pan to the heat and add the chicken stock. Bring the stock just to a boil and remove pan from heat.

4. Cover the pan and place it into the oven. Bake for 10–12 minutes until chops are almost cooked through. Remove the foil and bake for 5–7 minutes longer until chops spring back to the touch and most of the liquid is evaporated. Remove from the oven, cover loosely and allow the meat to rest before serving.

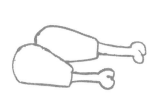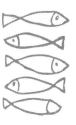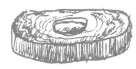

Caramelized Duck Breasts with Blueberries

Blueberries make the perfect compote to balance the robust flavor of duck. Serve the duck and compote over a bed of greens for a tasty salad.

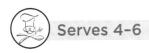 **Serves 4-6**

- 1 tbsp. coconut oil
- 1 tsp. minced shallot
- 1 ½ cups blueberries
- 1 tsp. lemon juice
- 2 (1 ¾- to 2-lb.) boneless Muscovy duck breasts, cut into four sides

1. Heat the coconut oil in a small saucepan over medium heat. Add the shallot and cook until just softened, about 2–3 minutes. Stir in the blueberries and lemon juice. Lower the heat to barely a simmer. Stir the mixture until the blueberries start to juice, about 3–4 minutes. Stir 2–3 minutes longer until fruit has popped and mixture is slightly juicy. Remove from heat and keep warm.

2. Heat two large skillets over high heat. Prick the skin of the ducks breasts all over with a fork without piercing the meat. Place the breasts skin side down in the hot skillets. Lower the heat to medium-high. Every 4–5 minutes, turn the breasts and prick the skin all over. Flip back over. Drain off any excess fat and reserve for future use if desired. Continue cooking and turning to prick skins until most of the fat has rendered from under the skin and the skin is crisp and golden, about 10 minutes. Turn and cook the other side of the breast for 3–4 minutes for medium rare (5–8 minutes longer for medium or well done). Remove from the heat and cover with foil to let rest for 8–10 minutes.

3. To serve, thinly slice the duck breasts and serve with the warm blueberry sauce.

Chef's Tip: D'Artagnan and Grimaud Farms both produce a free range duck. Muscovy ducks have leaner meat than Pekin ducks and a mildly gamey flavor. Duck fat has a high smoke point and may be frozen.

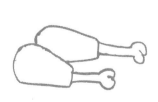
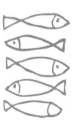
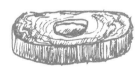

Codfish with Dill

This recipe is excellent for any thick white fish like halibut or hake.

 Serves 4

- 1 tbsp. coconut oil
- ¼ cup Mayonnaise (see recipe p. 54)
- 1 tsp. ground mustard
- 2 tbsps. lemon juice
- 2 scallions, trimmed and coarsely chopped
- ½ tsp. cayenne pepper
- 2 tsps. chopped dill
- 4 (6-oz.) cod filets
- Freshly ground black pepper to taste
- ¼ cup almond meal

1. Preheat the broiler on high. Lightly grease a baking sheet with the coconut oil and set aside.

2. In a medium bowl, whisk together the mayonnaise, mustard and lemon juice. Stir in the scallions, cayenne pepper and chopped dill.

3. Arrange the cod on the baking sheet. Season with freshly ground black pepper. Divide the mayonnaise mixture among the four filets, spreading the tops to coat evenly. Place the fish under the broiler and cook for 6–8 minutes, until fish flakes easily and is cooked through. Sprinkle the almond meal evenly over the filets and broil 1–2 minutes longer, until just browned. Remove from oven and serve immediately.

Halibut with Zucchini and Scallions

A simple preparation of halibut is all that is needed to bring out the flavor in this robust fish.

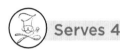 **Serves 4**

- 4 tbsps. extra virgin olive oil
- 6 scallions, ends trimmed and coarsely chopped
- 2 small zucchini, ends trimmed and cut into ¼-inch dice
- ½ tsp. minced garlic
- 2 tsps. chopped fresh thyme
- 4 (6-oz.) halibut filets
- Freshly ground pepper to taste
- 2 tsps. lemon juice

1. Heat 2 tbsps. olive oil in a medium skillet over medium-high heat. Add the scallions and cook for 2 minutes. Add the zucchini and cook for 4–5 minutes longer, until tender. Add the garlic and cook for 1 minute longer. Remove from heat and stir in the thyme. Keep warm.

2. Heat the remaining 2 tbsps. olive oil in a large skillet over medium-high heat. Season the filets with freshly ground pepper and add to the pan. Cook for 4–5 minutes, until just browned. Turn the fish and cook for 3–4 minutes longer, until just cooked through. Sprinkle the lemon juice evenly over the filets. Divide the vegetables among the fish filets to serve.

Salmon with Sweet Onions, Mustard and Rosemary

In this dish, salmon is roasted in the oven, but feel free to take advantage of an outdoor grill for cooking. Grilling the salmon on a well soaked alder plank adds additional flavor to the fish.

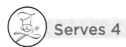 Serves 4

- 3 tbsps. extra virgin olive oil
- 1 tsp. ground mustard
- 2 tsps. lemon juice
- 1 tsp. chopped fresh rosemary
- 1 cup sliced sweet onions
- 4 (6-oz.) salmon filets
- Freshly ground pepper to taste

1. Preheat the oven to 325 degrees F. Lightly grease a baking sheet or roasting pan with 1 tbsp. olive oil and set aside.

2. In a medium bowl, whisk together the remaining 2 tbsps. olive oil, mustard and lemon juice. Stir in the rosemary. Add the onions and toss to coat.

3. Place the salmon skin side down onto the baking sheet. Season the filets with pepper. Divide the onion mixture evenly among the salmon pieces, mounding the onions on top. Bake for 20–25 minutes until the salmon flakes easily and the onions are cooked through and their edges begin to brown.

Braised Veal Shanks

This Paleo version of the Italian classic Osso Bucco is well worth the time it takes to prepare. Having your ingredients measured ahead of time will ease the preparation.

 Serves 4

- 3 tbsps. chopped fresh flat-leaf parsley
- 2 tbsps. freshly grated lemon zest
- 3 tsps. minced garlic
- Freshly ground black pepper
- 2 tbsps. almond flour
- 3 tbsps. extra virgin olive oil
- 4 (1 ¼-inch thick) veal shanks
- 1 cup chopped onion

- ¼ cup chopped carrot
- ¼ cup chopped celery
- ½ cup dry white wine (optional)
- 2 cups Chicken Stock (see Recipe p. 42)
- 1 tbsp. chopped basil
- 1 bay leaf
- 2 sprigs fresh thyme

1. Preheat the oven to 350 degrees F.

2. In a small bowl, combine the parsley, lemon zest and 2 tsps. minced garlic. Season with freshly ground pepper, cover and refrigerate until ready to use.

3. Tie a piece of butcher's twine around each of the veal shanks to hold the meat onto the bone. Season with freshly ground pepper and sprinkle the almond flour evenly over them.

4. Heat 2 tbsps. oil in a Dutch oven over medium-high heat. Add the veal to the pan. Cook for 4–5 minutes until browned. Turn the shanks and cook for 3–4 minutes longer. Transfer veal to a plate and cover to keep warm. Add the remaining oil to the pan and lower the heat to low. Add the remaining garlic, onion, carrot and celery and stir until beginning to soften, about 4–5 minutes. Raise the heat to medium-high. Stir in

wine (if using) or use 1/4 cup chicken stock, scraping off any bits of meat on the bottom, and cook until liquid is reduced in half, about 2 minutes. Add the chicken stock, basil, bay leaf and thyme and bring just to a boil. Reduce the heat to low and place the veal shanks back into the pan. Cover and place into the oven. Roast for 1 1/2-2 hours, until the veal is tender. Remove the pan from the oven and carefully remove the veal shanks onto a plate. Return the pan to the stove top over low heat and bring to a simmer. Remove and discard the bay leaf and thyme sprigs. Stir in half of the parsley mixture and allow sauce to thicken slightly, about 3–4 minutes. Cut the twine off the veal shanks and spoon on the sauce. Sprinkle the remaining parsley mixture evenly over the veal shanks to serve.

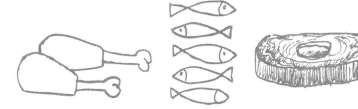

Trout with Lemon and Pine Nuts

The combination of paprika, sesame seeds and pine nuts adds a Moroccan flavor twist to a simple broiled trout.

 **Serves 4**

- 4 tbsps. extra virgin olive oil
- ¼ cup toasted pine nuts
- 1 tbsp. sesame seeds
- 2 tbsps. lemon juice
- 1 tsp. minced garlic

- 2 tbsps. freshly grated lemon zest
- ½ tsp. smoked paprika
- 2 tbsps. chopped dill
- 4 (6- to 8-oz.) trout filets
- Freshly ground pepper to taste

1. Preheat the broiler. Lightly grease a baking sheet with 1 tbsp. olive oil and set aside.

2. Divide the pine nuts in half. Coarsely chop half of the pine nuts and place into a small bowl. Toss together with the whole pine nuts, 2 tbsps. olive oil, sesame seeds, 1 tbsp. lemon juice, garlic, lemon zest, paprika and dill. Set aside.

3. Place the trout onto a baking sheet with the skin side down. Season the trout with the remaining olive oil, lemon juice and freshly ground pepper. Place under the broiler and cook until the fish flakes and is cooked through, about 5–6 minutes. Spoon pine nut topping evenly over fish to serve.

Sea Scallops with Green Curry and Zucchini

Any combination of seafood works well in this fresh green curry. Asian markets are an inexpensive source for Thai ingredients like kaffir lime leaves and lemon grass.

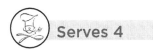 **Serves 4**

- 4 scallions, ends trimmed and coarsely chopped
- 3 tbsps. fresh chopped cilantro
- 2 kaffir lime leaves, finely chopped
- 4 Thai chili peppers, seeded and minced
- 1 lemon grass stalk, coarsely chopped
- 2 tsps. grated fresh ginger
- 3 tbsps. coconut oil
- 2 medium zucchini, ends trimmed and cut into spaghetti-thin strips
- 16 large dry sea scallops
- 1 cup sliced onions
- 1 ½ cups coconut milk
- ¼ cup fresh basil leaves (Thai basil if available)
- 2 tbsps. lime juice
- Freshly ground black pepper to taste

1. Combine the scallions, cilantro, lime leaves, chili peppers, lemon grass and ginger in a food processor until smooth. Add 1 tbsp. coconut oil and pulse to combine.

2. Heat 1 tbsp. coconut oil in a skillet or wok over medium heat. Add the zucchini and sauté until softened, about 2–3 minutes. Remove from the pan into a large bowl and cover to keep warm.

3. Heat the remaining 1 tbsp. coconut oil in the pan. Add the scallops and cook for 4–5 minutes, until edges are beginning to brown. Turn the scallops over and cook for 1–2 minutes longer, until opaque and just cooked through. Remove the scallops to a plate and cover to keep warm.

4. Add the onions to the pan and stir for 1 minute. Pour in the coconut milk and bring to a boil. Lower to a simmer. Stir in the reserved green curry paste. Simmer until the milk thickens slightly and the onions are soft and cooked through, about 10 minutes. Stir in the basil leaves and lime juice. Season with black pepper to taste. Remove from heat and add the scallops. Pour over the zucchini to serve.

Chef's Tip: Dry scallops are not treated with a solution called STP (sodium tripolyphosphate), which helps the scallops maintain their moisture ((STP treated scallops may be labeled "wet" or may not be labeled at all). The STP solution gives scallops a longer shelf life and adds water weight (and cost). The excess moisture will prevent the scallops from browning. Ask specifically if the scallops are dry before purchasing.

Flank Steak with Cilantro and Mint

Inexpensive cuts of beef like flank steak benefit from a savory marinade and a quick sear on the grill or under the broiler.

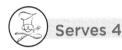 **Serves 4**

- 3 tbsps. lime juice
- 1 tsp. ground coriander
- 3 scallions, ends trimmed and coarsely chopped
- 2 tsps. fresh grated ginger
- 1 tsp. minced garlic
- ¼ cup extra virgin olive oil
- 1 ½–2 lbs. flank steak
- Freshly ground black pepper to taste
- 1 tbsp. chopped fresh cilantro
- 1 tbsp. chopped fresh mint

1. Combine the lime juice, coriander, scallions, ginger and garlic in a medium bowl. Divide the mixture in half. Whisk the olive oil into one half to make the marinade. Place the steak into a shallow bowl or Ziploc bag and pour the marinade over it. Marinate the meat in the refrigerator for 2–3 hours.

2. Pour the second half of the reserved mixture into a small saucepan and add 3 tbsps. water. Cook over medium heat until reduced by half and slightly thickened, about 4–5 minutes. Set aside.

3. Preheat the grill or broiler. Remove the meat and discard the marinade. Pat the meat dry and season with black pepper. Place the meat onto the grill (or in a roasting pan under the broiler) and cook for 6–7 minutes until brown. Turn the meat and cook 2–3 minutes longer for medium rare. Remove from the grill and allow the steak to rest for at least 5 minutes.

4. Reheat the sauce and stir in the cilantro and mint. Drizzle the steak with the sauce to serve.

Chef's Tip: Slice the flank steak on a 45-degree angle across the width or grain into thin strips for the most tender meat.

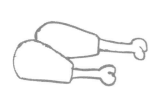 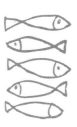 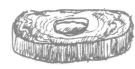

Salmon with Shitakes and Scallions

Cooking salmon in parchment yields a tender flavorful dish.

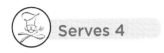 **Serves 4**

- 3 tbsps. avocado oil
- 1 cup sliced shitake mushrooms
- 4 scallions, ends trimmed and coarsely chopped
- 12 asparagus spears, ends trimmed and blanched
- 2 tbsps. lemon juice
- 4 (8-oz.) skinless salmon filets
- 2 tsps. chopped fresh dill

1. Preheat oven to 400 degrees F.

2. Fold four 12" x 16" parchment sheets in half to make a crease. Cut a half-circle starting at each crease. Then unfold to lay flat (shape will resemble a paper heart). Coat each piece of parchment with 1 tbsp. oil on both sides.

3. Toss the shitakes and scallions together in a medium bowl. Toss with the remaining avocado oil and lemon juice. Place 4 asparagus spears next to the crease on each piece of parchment. Place a piece of salmon on top. Evenly divide the mushroom mixture over the 4 filets. Season with freshly ground black pepper. Fold the other half circle over and fold the edges to seal. Fold the last crease in the opposite direction of the rest to ensure it seals. Repeat with remaining 3 pouches. Place pouches onto a baking sheet.

4. Bake for 15 minutes. Remove from oven and allow to rest for 5 minutes before cutting open parchment. Sprinkle with fresh dill to serve.

Rack of Lamb with Mint Pesto and Pecans

Flavorful lamb racks are roasted with a mint and pecan crust for a quick yet elegant dish.

 Serves 4

- 2 cups fresh mint leaves
- 1 tsp. minced garlic
- ¼ cup plus 2 tbsps. extra virgin olive oil

- 2 lamb racks (8 ribs per rack), trimmed of excess fat and bones cleaned
- Freshly ground pepper to taste
- ¼ cup coarsely ground pecans

1. Preheat the oven to 425 degrees F.

2. Combine the mint, garlic and 1/4 cup olive oil in a food processor and process until smooth. Set aside.

3. Brush 2 tbsps. olive oil over the lamb and wrap the bones in aluminum foil. Season the lamb with black pepper. Place the racks meat side down in a shallow roasting pan. Roast the lamb for 10–12 minutes for medium rare (4–8 minutes longer for medium to well done). Turn the lamb over and spread on the mint pesto. Press on the ground pecans and return pan to oven. Roast for 4 minutes longer, until the crust is lightly browned. Cover loosely with foil and allow the lamb to rest for 5 minutes before removing the foil from the ribs and cutting to serve.

Venison Medallions with Apple, Pear and Cranberries

The apple and pear acts to balance the tartness of the cranberries in this savory compote. Venison tenderloins from New Zealand have a deep burgundy color and rich flavor. The tenderloin is a delicate cut and is best cooked briefly to preserve the tenderness.

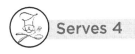 Serves 4

- ½ cup cranberries
- 1 sweet apple such as Fuji or Gala, peeled and finely chopped
- 2 tsps. lemon juice
- 2 large ripe pears, peeled and coarsely chopped
- 1 sprig thyme
- 2 venison tenderloins
- Freshly ground pepper to taste
- 2 tbsps. almond flour
- 3 tbsps. extra virgin olive oil
- ½ cup coconut milk

1. Combine cranberries, apple, 1/2 cup water and lemon juice in a medium saucepan over medium-high heat. When cranberries begin to pop, reduce heat to medium-low and stir in the pears and thyme. Cover and gently simmer, stirring occasionally, until the pears are very tender, about 12–15 minutes. Remove and discard the thyme. Set aside until ready to serve.

2. Trim off the ends of the tenderloins and slice the remaining pieces into 2-inch-thick medallions. Pound each piece to flatten it slightly. Season the medallions with pepper and dredge lightly in the flour. Heat the olive oil in a large skillet over medium-high heat. Add the venison and cook until browned but still medium rare in the center, about 2 minutes per side (2–4 minutes longer for medium to well done). Keep warm. Add the coconut milk to the skillet and scrape any bits of meat off the bottom of the pan. Reduce the milk in half and remove from heat. Add the venison and any juices back into the skillet and turn the pieces to coat with the sauce. Serve venison with warm compote.

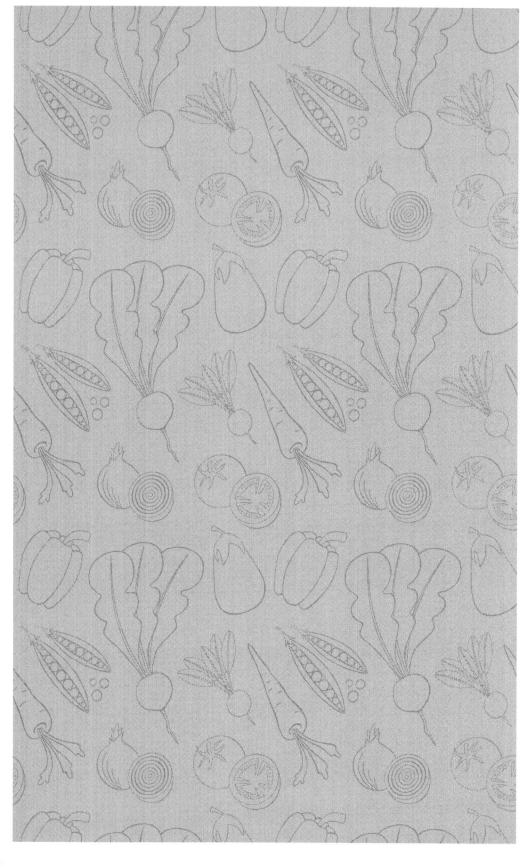

Chapter 8

Sides

- Pumpkin with Caramelized Shallots and Walnuts
- Roasted Brussels Sprouts
- Carrot, Sweet Potato and Parsnip Oven Fries
- Mixed Cabbage and Carrot Slaw
- Beet Greens with Onions and Walnuts
- Celery Root and Turnip Puree
- Creamy Shredded Pumpkin
- Braised Swiss Chard and Kale
- Roasted Summer Vegetables

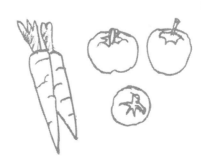

Pumpkin with Caramelized Shallots and Walnuts

Roasted pumpkin is a delicious accompaniment to roasted pork, chicken and turkey.

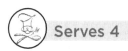 **Serves 4**

- 1 small pie pumpkin (about 5–6 lbs.), rinsed and patted dry
- 3 tbsps. extra virgin olive oil
- 1 tsp. freshly grated nutmeg
- 1 tsp. ground allspice
- 1 tsp. ground ginger
- 2 small shallots, peeled and thinly sliced into rings
- ½ cup toasted walnuts

1. Preheat the oven to 400 degrees F. Line a baking sheet with parchment or aluminum foil.

2. Slice the pumpkin in half from top to bottom. Remove the stem and discard. Scrape out the seeds and save for another use or discard. Cut the pumpkin into 1/2-inch-thick slices. Place the slices in a large bowl. Toss with 2 tbsps. olive oil, nutmeg, all spice and ginger. Lay the slices onto the baking sheet and place into the oven. Roast for 20–25 minutes until the edges begin to brown and the flesh is tender. Remove from the oven and allow to cool slightly.

3. Heat the remaining olive oil in a medium skillet over medium heat. Add the shallots and sauté, stirring constantly, until soft and golden, about 6–8 minutes. Spoon the shallots evenly over the pumpkin slices and sprinkle with the walnuts to serve.

Chef's Tip: The pumpkin seeds may be toasted for a delicious snack. Preheat the oven to 300 degrees F. Rinse and dry the seeds and spread them out on a lightly greased baking sheet. Toast, stirring every 10 minutes, for about 40 minutes until golden brown. The seeds may be tossed with paprika, chili powder or other savory seasonings before toasting.

Roasted Brussels Sprouts

Roasting Brussels sprouts adds a nutty, caramelized flavor. The addition of nuts adds texture to this simply delicious dish.

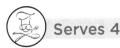 **Serves 4**

- 1 ½ lbs. Brussels sprouts
- 3 tbsps. extra virgin olive oil
- 2 tsps. freshly squeezed lemon juice
- 1 tsp. smoked paprika
- ½ tsp. freshly ground black pepper
- ½ cup toasted pecans or walnuts, coarsely chopped

1. Preheat oven to 400 degrees F.

2. Cut off the brown ends of the Brussels sprouts. Slice the Brussels sprouts in half from top to bottom. Mix them in a bowl with the olive oil, lemon juice, paprika and pepper. Pour them onto a sheet pan and roast for 35 to 40 minutes, until crisp on the outside and tender on the inside. Shake the pan from time to time to brown the sprouts evenly. Sprinkle with more freshly ground pepper to taste.

Carrot, Sweet Potato and Parsnip Oven Fries

Oven-roasted sweet potatoes, carrots and parsnips make a delicious alternative to traditional potato fries.

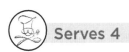 **Serves 4**

- 4 tbsps. extra virgin olive oil
- 2 sweet potatoes, peeled
- 5 medium carrots, peeled and ends trimmed

- 3 medium parsnips, peeled and ends trimmed
- ½ teaspoon freshly ground black pepper
- 1 tsp. crushed red pepper flakes

1. Preheat oven to 400 degrees F. Lightly grease a rimmed baking sheet with 1 tbsp. olive oil and set aside.

2. Cut the potatoes lengthwise into 1/4-inch-thick disks, then cut these disks lengthwise into 1/4-inch-thick sticks. Trim as necessary to keep the slices a uniform size. Slice the carrots and parsnips lengthwise into 1/4-inch-thick planks. Slice lengthwise again to make 1/4-inch-thick fries.

3. Place the cut vegetables into a large bowl and toss with the remaining 3 tbsps. of oil, black pepper and red pepper flakes. Spread into a single layer and roast for 10 minutes. Flip the vegetables and cook for 10–15 minutes longer, until crisp and golden brown.

Mixed Cabbage and Carrot Slaw

This Asian inspired slaw is an interesting Paleo variation on traditional coleslaw with mayonnaise.

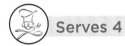 Serves 4

- 3 tbsps. lime juice
- 1 tbsp. toasted sesame oil
- ½ cup avocado oil
- 1 ½ tsps. grated fresh ginger
- 1 tsp. minced garlic
- 2 red Thai chili peppers, seeded and minced
- ½ tsp. crushed red pepperflakes

- 4 cups shredded Napa cabbage
- 1 cup shredded red cabbage
- 1 cup shredded carrots
- 4 scallions, trimmed and thinly sliced
- ¼ cup fresh chopped cilantro
- 1 avocado, peeled, pitted and cut into ¼-inch chunks

1. Freshly ground pepper to taste

2. Whisk together the lime juice, sesame oil, avocado oil, ginger, garlic, peppers and pepper flakes in a large bowl. Add the Napa cabbage, red cabbage, carrots, scallions and cilantro and toss to combine. Cover and refrigerate for 1 hour to allow flavors to blend. When ready to serve, add the avocado and toss to combine. Season with pepper to taste.

Beet Greens with Onions and Walnuts

Kale or Swiss chard will work equally well in this tasty side dish. Add some strips of grilled pork or chicken for a simple, delicious dinner.

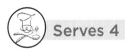 Serves 4

- 2 tbsps. extra virgin olive oil
- 1 ½ cups sliced red onion
- 1 tsp. minced garlic
- 8–10 cups stemmed beet greens

- ½ cup Chicken Stock (see Recipe p. 42)
- 2 tsps. lemon juice
- 1 tsp. crushed red pepper flakes
- ¼ cup coarsely chopped walnuts

1. Freshly ground black pepper to taste

2. Heat the olive oil in a large skillet over medium-high heat. Add the onion and cook until softened, about 4–5 minutes. Add the garlic and cook 30 seconds longer. Stir in the beet greens. Add the chicken stock and bring to a simmer (add extra stock if necessary to just cover the greens). Lower the heat to a simmer and cook until the greens are tender, about 4–6 minutes. Remove from the heat and drain any excess liquid. Stir in the lemon juice and pepper flakes. Sprinkle with walnuts and season with freshly ground pepper to serve.

Celery Root and Turnip Puree

Also known as celeriac, celery root is a type of celery cultivated for its edible albeit gnarly root. It's not always available, so when you see it, buy some. If you miss traditional mashed potatoes, this puree will make you a satisfied Paleo eater.

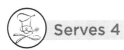 **Serves 4**

- 2 cups coconut milk
- 1 cup Chicken Stock (see Recipe p. 42)
- 1 lb. celery root, peeled and coarsely chopped (about 2 cups)
- 1 lb. medium turnips, peeled and coarsely chopped (about 3 cups)
- 2 tbsps. coconut oil
- ¼ tsp. cayenne pepper
- 1 tsp. chopped flat-leaf parsley

1. Pour coconut milk into a large saucepan. Stir in the chicken stock and 1 cup of water. Add celery root and turnip and bring to a boil. Lower the heat and simmer until tender, about 20–25 minutes. Pour off excess liquid.

2. Place the vegetables into the food processor. Puree until smooth. Add the coconut oil, cayenne pepper and parsley and pulse just to combine, then serve.

Chef's Tip: If celery root is unavailable, the turnips alone are also quite delicious. Just double the amount of turnips and follow the same recipe.

Creamy Shredded Pumpkin

This is a delicious accompaniment to game entrees like rabbit or venison. Shredding pumpkin is a great way to add texture.

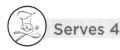 **Serves 4**

- 2 tbsps. coconut oil
- 1 tsp. chopped shallot
- 3 cups fresh shredded pumpkin (see note below)
- 1 cup coconut milk

- 1 tsp. freshly grated nutmeg
- ½ tsp. chopped thyme
- ½ tsp. chopped sage
- ½ cup slivered almonds (optional)

- In a large skillet, melt the coconut oil over medium-high heat. Add the shallot and cook until softened, about 1–2 minutes. Add the fresh pumpkin and sauté for 2–3 minutes. Add the coconut milk and lower heat to a simmer. Stir in the nutmeg, thyme and sage. Allow the mixture to simmer over low heat until the pumpkin is tender and the milk has thickened, about 10–12 minutes. Remove from heat and stir in the almonds (if desired), then serve.

Chef's Tip: Here is how to shred fresh pumpkin. Select a smaller "pie" pumpkin. Cut a wide circle around the stem through the flesh and remove and discard the top piece. Scoop out the insides (reserve seeds for toasting if desired). Cut the pumpkin into quarters. Cut each quarter again into half. Remove the skin with a knife or vegetable peeler. Use a box grater or food processor to shred the pumpkin.

Braised Swiss Chard and Kale

Swiss chard and kale are a dynamic duo of healthy greens featuring an amazing array of phytonutrients and antioxidants.

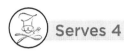 **Serves 4**

- 3 tbsps. extra virgin olive oil
- 1 cup sliced onion
- 3 cloves garlic, peeled and thinly sliced
- 2 tsps. ground cumin
- 1 tsp. crushed red pepper flakes
- 1 bunch Swiss chard, stems thinly sliced and leaves cut into 1-inch ribbons (about 4 cups)
- 1 bunch kale, stems removed and leaves cut into 1-inch ribbons (about 4 cups)
- 1 tart apple (such as Granny Smith), peeled, seeded and diced
- 1 ½ cups Chicken Stock (see Recipe p. 42)
- Freshly ground pepper
- 2 tsps. lemon juice

- In a large skillet or Dutch oven, heat the oil over medium heat. Add the onion, garlic, cumin and red pepper flakes. Sauté until the onion is softened, about 4–5 minutes. Add the chard and kale. Cook, stirring, until the leaves are wilted. Add the apple. Add the stock and bring to a boil. Lower to a simmer and cover, stirring every few minutes. Cook until the stems are tender, about 6–8 minutes. Season with freshly ground pepper and stir in lemon juice to serve.

Roasted Summer Vegetables

A simple preparation yields delicious results for fresh summer vegetables.

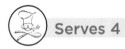 **Serves 4**

- 4 tbsps. extra virgin olive oil
- 1 tsp. chopped garlic
- 1 shallot, peeled and minced
- 2 tsps. chopped fresh thyme
- 2 tsps. lemon zest
- 2 tbsps. lemon juice
- Freshly ground pepper to taste
- 2 medium zucchini, sliced into thin rounds
- 1 medium summer squash, sliced into thin rounds
- 1 Japanese eggplant, sliced into thin rounds
- 3 plum tomatoes, sliced into thin rounds
- 3 tbsps. chopped flat-leaf parsley

1. Preheat the oven to 400 degrees F. Lightly grease an oval or square 1 1/2–2-qt. baking dish with 1 tbsp. olive oil and set aside.

2. In a medium skillet, heat 3 tbsps. olive oil over medium heat. Add the garlic and shallot and cook for 30 seconds. Remove from heat and stir in the thyme, lemon zest and 1 tbsp. lemon juice. Toss the zucchini, squash and eggplant slices with the oil to coat evenly.

3. Arrange overlapping slices of squash, eggplant and tomato in the prepared baking dish. Bake until the vegetables are lightly browned and tender, about 35–40 minutes. Sprinkle with the remaining lemon juice and parsley to serve.

Chapter 9

Drinks and Desserts

- Watermelon Mint Agua Fresca
- Cucumber Basil Water
- Blueberry Peach Smoothie
- Cantaloupe Banana Smoothie
- Strawberry Sorbet with Basil
- Melon Mint Granita
- Apple Spice Granita
- Pumpkin Custard
- Coconut Soufflé with Pineapple and Kiwi
- Key Lime and Mango Ice Cream
- Strawberry Banana Ice Cream
- Roasted Pears with Almond Crumble
- Banana Custard with Coconut and Macadamia Nuts
- Cherry Crisp
- Mango and Pineapple with Coconut Cream and Cashews
- Mint Berry Cream

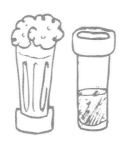

Watermelon Mint Agua Fresca

Agua fresca, literally Spanish for "fresh water," is a light, non-alcoholic drink served by street vendors, in bars and at eateries throughout Central America, Mexico and the Caribbean. This version leaves out any sweetener for a Paleo-friendly beverage.

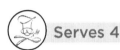 **Serves 4**

- 4 cups seedless watermelon, cut into large chunks
- 2 teaspoons lime juice
- 8 fresh mint leaves for muddling
- 4 lime slices for garnish (if desired)

- In a food processor or blender, process half the watermelon pieces with 1 cup of water until smooth. Pour into a pitcher. Repeat the process with the remaining melon and water. Stir in the lime juice. Place two mint leaves into each glass. Place the muddler (or use a wooden spoon) into the glass and press down with it lightly on the leaves about 5–6 times (the purpose is to release the oils in the mint, not to pulverize it). Add ice and fill each glass with the watermelon mixture. Garnish with lime slices (if desired) and serve.

Variation: Substitute 4 cups mango (about three large mangos, peeled and seeded) or 4 cups pineapple for the watermelon.

Cucumber Basil Water

Cucumbers contain antioxidants and have anti-inflammatory qualities. Combined with lemon and water – they make a delicious, refreshing alternative to processed drinks.

 Serves 4

- 4 ½ cups coarsely chopped, seeded, peeled cucumbers (about 4 medium size cucumbers)
- ⅓ cup fresh lemon juice
- 8 fresh basil leaves for muddling
- 4 lemon slices for garnish if desired

- In a food processor or blender, combine half of the cucumber with 1 cup cold water until smooth. Pour into a pitcher. Repeat the process with the remaining cucumber and water. Stir in the lemon juice. Place two basil leaves in each glass. Place the muddler (or use a wooden spoon) into the glass and press down with it lightly on the leaves about 5 6 times (the purpose is to release the oils in the basil, not to pulverize it). Add ice and fill each glass with the cucumber mixture. Garnish with lemon slices (if desired) and serve.

Blueberry Peach Smoothie

Blueberries and juicy peaches combine for a creamy treat.

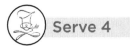 **Serve 4**

- 6 peaches, peeled, pitted and chopped
- 2 cups blueberries

- 2 cups coconut milk
- 1 tsp. cinnamon
- 1 tsp. lemon juice

- Combine all ingredients together in a blender until smooth.

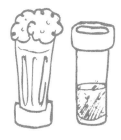

Cantaloupe Banana Smoothie

Bananas give a creamy consistency to this summer drink.

 Serves 4

- 1 medium cantaloupe, rind removed, seeded and cut into chunks (about 4 cups)
- 2 medium bananas, peeled and sliced

- 2 tsps. lemon juice
- 1 cup coconut milk

- Place peaches, cantaloupe, banana and lemon juice into a blender and process until smooth. Add coconut milk and blend until smooth. Add extra coconut milk as necessary if a thinner consistency is desired.

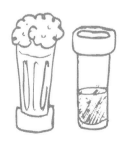

Strawberry Sorbet with Basil

You won't taste the apple but it will supply a little added sweetness to this summery sorbet.

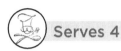 **Serves 4**

- 1 quart fresh strawberries, hulled
- 1 sweet apple (such as Fuji or Red Delicious), peeled, seeded and chopped
- 2 tsps. lemon juice
- ¼ cup fresh basil leaves

1. Place the strawberries, apple and lemon juice into a food processor or blender and pulse just to combine. Allow the mixture to sit for about 30 minutes. Add the fresh basil and pulse to combine. Finishing processing the mixture until it's smooth.

2. Freeze the mixture in an ice cream freezer according to manufacturer's instructions for at least 30 minutes (or follow instructions on p. 38 for processing without a machine). If you would like the mixture harder after this, remove it from the container and spoon it into a lidded container. Freeze at least 1 hour longer before serving.

Melon Mint Granita

Granitas are a coarse Italian-style frozen dessert. This granita uses sweet ripe melon for flavor and pureed apples for sweetness. Lime juice and the addition of chopped mint perks up the flavors. For a dramatic presentation, garnish with whole blackberries and mint leaves.

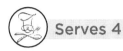 **Serves 4**

- 4 cups honeydew, peeled, seeded and cubed
- 1 sweet apple, peeled, seeded and chopped coarsely
- ¼ cup lime juice
- 1 tsp. finely chopped mint
- 1 cup fresh blackberries, for garnish
- Fresh mint leaves, for garnish

1. Place a 9" x 13" baking sheet (or metal pan) into the freezer and chill for at least 30 minutes.

2. With a food processor or blender, combine melon, apple and lime juice until smooth. Add the chopped mint and pulse until just combined. Pour the mixture evenly into the chilled pan.

3. Place the pan on a level surface in your freezer. Chill until ice crystals begin to from around edges, about 30 minutes. Remove the pan from the freezer and stir the mixture with a fork to incorporate all the crystals. Continue freezing and then stirring every 30 minutes, moving the frozen edges in toward the slushy center and crushing any lumps until frozen but not solid, about 3–4 hours. Spoon the crystals into a Ziploc bag or container with lid and freeze until ready to serve.

4. Remove from the freezer about 20 minutes before serving to soften slightly. Sprinkle with blackberries and garnish with mint leaves, if desired.

Chef's Tip: The key to a good texture is to be consistent in the scraping of the crystals with a fork.

Apple Spice Granita

A tasty frozen ice dessert made with sweet apples and spices.

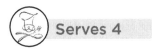 **Serves 4**

- 4 cups sweet apples (such as Fuji or Gala), peeled, seeded and coarsely chopped
- 1 ½ tbsps. lemon juice

- ½ tsp. ground cinnamon
- ¼ tsp. grated nutmeg
- ¼ tsp. ground clove

1. Place a 9" x 13" inch baking sheet (or metal pan) into the freezer and chill for at least 30 minutes.

2. In a food processor or blender, combine all of the ingredients until smooth. Pour the mixture evenly into the chilled pan. Place the pan on a level surface in the freezer. Chill until ice crystals begin to from around edges, about 30 minutes. Remove the pan from the freezer and stir the mixture with a fork to incorporate all the crystals. Continue freezing and then stirring every 30 minutes, moving the frozen edges in toward the slushy center and crushing any lumps until frozen but not solid, about 3–4 hours. Spoon the crystals into a Ziploc bag or container with lid and freeze until ready to serve.

3. Remove from the freezer about 20 minutes before serving to soften slightly.

Pumpkin Custard

These individual custards are reminiscent of pumpkin pie without the addition of sugar. Chopped apples add a little sweetness to the finished custard. They also make a delicious savory side dish without the apples.

 Serves 4

- 1–2 tbsps. coconut oil
- 1 ½ cups pumpkin puree
- 3 eggs
- ½ cup coconut milk

- 2 tsps. cinnamon
- 1 tsp. nutmeg
- ¼ tsp. ground cloves
- 1 cup coarsely chopped sweet apples, such as Fuji or Gala

1. Preheat the oven to 350 degrees F. Lightly grease 4 individual 5- to 6-oz. ramekins with the coconut oil.

2. In a large bowl, whisk together the pumpkin puree and eggs. Add the coconut milk and stir to combine. Stir in the cinnamon, nutmeg and cloves. Divide the mixture among the 4 ramekins. Place ramekins in a baking pan. Fill the pan with very hot water halfway up the sides of the cups.

3. Bake for 45–50 minutes, until lightly browned and centers are firm and cooked through. Allow to cool slightly. Divide apples evenly among the centers of the custards to serve.

Coconut Soufflé with Pineapple and Kiwi

Pineapple and kiwi add a hint of sweetness to this sophisticated Paleo dessert.

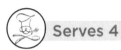 **Serves 4**

- 1 cup fresh pineapple chunks
- 1 tsp. lime juice
- 1–2 tbsps. coconut oil
- 2 tbsps. unsweetened shredded coconut
- 1 cup coconut milk
- 1 tbsp. almond meal
- 2 tbsps. coconut flour
- 3 egg yolks
- 1 tsp. vanilla extract
- 6 egg whites
- 2 small ripe kiwi, peeled and coarsely chopped
- ¼ cup coconut cream, whipped to soft peaks

1. In a food processor or blender, puree the pineapple with the lime juice. Set aside.

2. Preheat the oven to 375 degrees F. Lightly grease 4 individual 5- to 6-oz. ramekins with the oil. Sprinkle the inside with the shredded coconut to coat, tilting to evenly distribute. Tap out any excess and reserve for garnish if desired. Place ramekins onto a baking sheet.

3. Heat the coconut milk in a small saucepan over medium heat until steaming. Whisk in the almond meal and coconut flour and cook until slightly thickened, about 4–5 minutes. Whisk the egg yolks in a large bowl and slowly pour the coconut milk mixture over them. Whisk continuously until well combined. Stir in the vanilla extract.

4. Beat the egg whites in the bowl with an electric mixer on medium speed until shiny and stiff. Stir one-third of the whites into the

coconut/egg yolk mixture to lighten it. Gently fold in the remaining egg whites just until evenly distributed. Spoon the batter into the prepared dishes.

5. Bake until puffed and firm to the touch, about 10–12 minutes. Spoon the pineapple puree into the center of each soufflé. Evenly divide the kiwi and coconut cream among the 4 ramekins to serve.

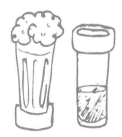

Key Lime and Mango Ice Cream

Sweet ripe mangos lend a creamy texture to this dairy-free dessert.

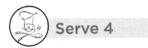 **Serve 4**

- 3 medium ripe mangos, peeled, seeded and cut into chunks
- 2 cups coconut milk
- ½ cup key lime juice

1. Place all ingredients into a blender or food processor and blend until smooth.

2. Pour the mixture into an ice cream maker and process according to the manufacturer's directions (or follow instructions on p. 38 for processing without a machine) for approximately 25–35 minutes. Serve as is for soft serve or freeze for another 3–4 hours to allow the ice cream to harden.

Chef's Tip: Substitute regular lime juice if key limes are unavailable.

Strawberry Banana Ice Cream

Bananas lend the creamy texture to this Paleo-friendly ice cream treat.

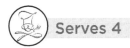 Serves 4

- 2 cups strawberries, hulled and sliced
- 2 medium bananas, very ripe, sliced
- 1 cup chopped sweet apple
- 2 cups coconut milk
- ¼ cup lemon juice
- ½ cup sliced almonds (optional)

1. Place all ingredients into a blender or food processor and blend until smooth.

2. Pour the mixture into an ice cream maker and process according to the manufacturer's directions (or follow instructions on p. 38 for processing without a machine) for approximately 25–35 minutes. In the last 5 minutes, stir in the almonds (if using). Serve as is for soft serve or freeze for another 3–4 hours to allow the ice cream to harden.

Chef's Tip: Layer this ice cream with fresh sliced strawberries and bananas in parfaits or popsicle molds and top with almonds for a dramatic presentation.

Roasted Pears with Almond Crumble

Sweet ripe pears baked with spices are topped with a crumbled topping in this easy-to-prepare dessert.

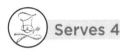 **Serves 4**

- 4 tbsps. coconut oil
- ¼ cup coconut flour
- 1 large egg
- 1 tsp. almond extract
- 3 tbsps. sliced almonds
- 4 small ripe pears, halved and cored
-

- ½ tsp. ground cinnamon
- ¼ tsp. ground clove
- 1 tsp. vanilla extract
- ¼ cup coconut cream, whipped to soft peaks (optional)

1. Preheat the oven to 375 degrees F. Lightly grease an 8" x 8" baking dish with 1 tbsp. oil and set aside.

2. In a medium bowl, combine 1 tbsp. coconut oil with the coconut flour. Stir in the egg and almond extract until completely combined. Stir in the toasted almonds and set aside.

3. Place the pears cut side down into the baking dish. Dot the tops of the pears with 2 tbsps. coconut oil. In a small bowl, whisk together 3 tbsps. water with the cinnamon, clove and vanilla extract. Pour the water mixture into the baking dish. Bake pears for 20–25 minutes until slightly tender.

4. Turn pears over and evenly divide the almond mixture over the pears. Return the pears to the oven and bake for 10–15 minutes longer, until mixture is lightly browned and pears are soft. Serve warm with coconut cream if desired.

Banana Custard with Coconut and Macadamia Nuts

This creamy banana custard may be layered in individual parfait glasses for a lovely presentation.

 Serves 4

- 3 ripe bananas
- 1 ½ cups coconut milk
- ¼ tsp. ground cinnamon
- 3 large egg yolks, beaten
- 1 teaspoon vanilla
- ¼ cup coconut cream
- ½ cup coarsely chopped macadamia nuts
- ¼ cup toasted coconut

1. Peel 2 bananas, cut into chunks and place into a medium bowl. Mash the bananas into a paste. In a small saucepan, heat the coconut milk just to a simmer. Remove from heat and whisk in the cinnamon.

2. In a medium size bowl, whisk the egg yolks with the vanilla. Temper the egg yolks by adding a small amount of hot milk, then gradually stir in the remaining milk. Pour the mixture into the saucepan and cook until thickened, then remove from heat. Stir in the mashed bananas. Spoon mixture into a bowl. Cover and chill custard for at least 1 hour.

3. To serve, whip the coconut cream to soft peaks. Peel the remaining banana and cut into thin slices. Fold the slices into the custard. Top custard with whipped cream of coconut. Combine the macadamia nuts and coconut in a small bowl. Sprinkle evenly over the custard to serve.

Cherry Crisp

Substitute any ripe fruit like berries or peaches for a seasonal variation of this delicious crisp.

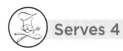 **Serves 4**

- 2–3 tbsps. coconut oil
- 4 cups ripe cherries, pitted and cut in half
- 1 tbsp. lemon juice
- ¼ cup coconut flour

- 1 large egg
- 1 tsp. almond extract
- 1 tbsp. sliced almonds
- 1 tbsp. large coconut flakes

1. Preheat the oven to 375 degrees F. Brush 4 individual 5- to 6-oz. ramekins with 1–2 tbsps. coconut oil. Toss the cherries with the lemon juice and fill each ramekin to the top. Dot the top of the cherries with 1 tbsp. coconut oil. Place onto a baking sheet and bake for 10–12 minutes, until fruit begins to bubble.

2. In the meantime, cut 1 tbsp. coconut oil into the flour in a medium bowl until crumbly. Stir in the egg and almond extract until mixture is combined. Stir in the almonds and coconut flakes. (Topping should be crumbly but not dry – add a little water as necessary to correct texture). Remove the cherries from the oven and crumble on the topping. Return to the oven and bake for 10–12 minutes longer or until the top is golden brown. Cool slightly to serve.

Chef's Tip: Mound the fruit high in the ramekins, as it will reduce in size as it cooks.

Mango and Pineapple with Coconut Cream and Cashews

Broiling (or grilling) mango and pineapple concentrates the sweetness and lightly caramelizes the edges for a lovely presentation.

 **Serves 4**

- 1 large mango, peeled, seeded and sliced lengthwise into ¼ -inch thick pieces
- 4 slices fresh pineapple, core removed

- 1 tsp. lime juice
- 1 cup coconut cream, whipped to soft peaks
- ½ cup coarsely chopped cashews
- 3 tbsps. coconut flakes

1. Preheat the broiler on high. Line 2 baking sheets with foil.

2. Arrange mango and pineapple slices in a single layer on the prepared pans. Broil the mango about 4 inches from the heat until browned in spots, 8–10 minutes. Broil the pineapple about 4 inches from the heat until edges begin to brown, 4–5 minutes. Sprinkle with the lime juice.

3. Serve the broiled fruit topped with coconut cream, cashews and coconut flakes.

Mint Berry Cream

This creamy base can also be processed in an ice cream maker for a frozen treat.

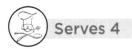 **Serves 4**

- 1 cup coconut cream
- ¼ cup mint leaves
- 1 tsp. vanilla extract
- 1 pint fresh strawberries, hulled and sliced

- 1 ½ cups fresh raspberries
- 1 tsp. lemon juice
- ½ cup fresh blackberries
- Mint sprigs for garnish (optional)

1. Heat the coconut cream in a small saucepan over medium heat until steaming. Remove from heat and stir in the mint leaves. Allow to steep until at room temperature, about 20 minutes. Strain out the mint and discard the leaves. Refrigerate the coconut milk until chilled, at least 1 hour.

2. Pour the chilled mint-infused coconut cream and vanilla into the food processor. Process until whipped and spoon into a bowl. Add half of the strawberries, 1 cup of the raspberries and the lemon juice to the processor bowl. Pulse until pureed. Whisk the pureed berries into the cream.

3. Mix the remaining berries together in a large bowl. Spoon the berry cream into individual serving bowls. Spoon the berries evenly over the dishes. Garnish with mint sprigs (if desired) to serve.

Chef's Tip: If you prefer to not have raspberry seeds in the cream base, process the raspberries in a food processor until pureed. Press the puree through a mesh sieve with the back of a spoon into a bowl. Discard the seeds and use the puree.

Special Bonus Offer to Say Thanks!

Thank you for purchasing this book. I am pleased to have you along for the journey to better health and better eating. I know you could have picked from dozens of cookbook about Paleo, so to show my appreciation, I'd like to offer you a bonus: *PALEO – Easy as 1-2-3 TEN GREAT GRILLING RECIPES*. Please go to my website www.donnaleahy.com (click here) - and sign up for my free newsletter. When we receive your confirmation, we'll email you the PDF. I will include you on my list for free recipes and tips and also periodically send you any exclusive special offerings as well. If you have a moment to review this book on Amazon (Click HERE), I'd really appreciate it. This kind of feedback will help me continue to write the kind of cookbooks that you want to use.

Thanks again and I look forward to hearing from you.

Index

Made in the USA
Lexington, KY
21 August 2014